Arthritis & Rheumatism

Symptoms, causes, orthodox treatment and how herbal medicine will help.

Other published and forthcoming titles in the series include:

IBS & Colitis

Menopause

Anxiety & Tension

Migraine & Headaches

Asthma & Bronchitis

Arthritis & Rheumatism

Jill Wright MNIMH

HERBAL HEALTH

Published in 2001 by
How To Books Ltd, 3 Newtec Place,
Magdalen Road, Oxford OX4 1RE, United Kingdom
Tel: (01865) 793806   Fax: (01865) 248780
email: info@howtobooks.co.uk
www.howtobooks.co.uk

British Library Cataloguing in Publication Data
A catalogue record for this book is available from
the British Library

Edited by Diana Brueton
Cover design by Shireen Nathoo Design, London
Produced for How To Books by Deer Park Productions
Designed and typeset by Shireen Nathoo Design, London
Printed and bound in Great Britain
by Bell & Bain Ltd., Glasgow

Note: The material contained in this book is set out in good
faith for general guidance and no liability can be accepted for
loss or expense incurred as a result of relying in particular
circumstances on statements made in the book. The laws and
regulations are complex and liable to change, and readers
should check the current position with the relevant authorities
before making personal arrangements.

Herbal Health *is an imprint of*
How To Books

Contents

Preface

Do you have deep aches in your muscles? Do you have one or more problem joints – stiff, clicky, swollen or painful? You could be developing arthritis and you may be able to do something about it, or you might already have been diagnosed with arthritis and/or rheumatism. By reading this book you can:

- Find out how you can prevent deterioration of the joints, relieve pain and improve mobility.

- Discover what herbal remedies can do to reduce inflammation and ease aching muscles without unpleasant side-effects.

- Learn how to combine herbs in the correct doses to achieve an individual prescription which will help your particular problems. A brief guide to how arthritis develops will help you to plan your own herbal prescription as well as understand your treatments and get more out of visits to doctors and consultants.

- Find out more about plant food as medicine, and how to maintain healthy bones and joints by eating the right foods.

Herbal medicine is the leading alternative to conventional treatment and is still the major form of medicine in many parts of the world. There are many advantages to using herbal remedies, and this book will guide you simply through the process of choosing the right one.

I am a member of the National Institute of Medical Herbalists, having trained for four years in herbal pharmacology, nutrition and medical sciences. I offer reliable, clear advice on the safe use of herbal medicines which will help to reduce symptoms and improve joint health. In this book I have written down the answers to questions which are frequently asked.

This advice is meant for general use only. If you have an allergy, or are taking any medication or have a medical condition which may affect your use of herbal medicine, you will need further help from a qualified practitioner. A list of useful addresses and websites is found in Sources and Resources at the end of the book.

Jill Wright

1

Understanding arthritis and rheumatism

All about bones, muscles and joints

Bones

Bone consists of a mesh or matrix of minerals – calcium, magnesium, phosphorus and carbon. These are all provided in the food we eat and we need to replace them each day as small quantities are lost during other body processes.

If we don't have enough of the essential minerals in our diet we may develop problems with the strength of our bones such as rickets, (or its adult version, osteomalacia). Most people associate calcium with bone strength, but vitamin D is required to ferry the calcium into our bones, therefore we must also have adequate daily amounts of this vitamin to ensure healthy bones. Our skin and kidneys make vitamin D using sunlight, but in a northern European climate we rely on dietary sources to help us out. More of these later.

The astonishing thing about bone is that it is constantly being made and unmade – by cells called osteoblasts (makers) and osteoclasts (breakers). This is how we are able to grow and repair the damage caused by falls and breaks. Sometimes, this process doesn't work properly and we suffer disorders such as osteoporosis. In osteoporosis, bone is 'eaten' away and not replaced, so that holes develop and it breaks more easily.

Muscles

Muscles are made of protein, arranged in bundles of fibres for strength. They use calcium, potassium and sodium to send and receive nerve impulses which enable them to work. They also use large amounts of sugar for fuel and this is stored in muscles ready for use in a special form called glycogen. Our adrenal hormones enable rapid use of this stored fuel when we need it, for example during exercise. There are two main benefits in regular exercise. We can increase the strength and bulk of muscles and exercise also sends messages to strengthen bones. On the other hand, lack of exercise lets muscles atrophy (shrink). The result is that they don't do such a good job in supporting joints – for example poor support for the vertebral column may result in back pain.

A lack of calcium or potassium may result in painful spasms known as cramp. Two sets of glands called the thyroid and the parathyroid, found in the neck, control the rate at which minerals are used in the body. A problem with either of these may lead to muscle cramps. Conditions such as kidney disease, which hastens the elimination of calcium and potassium from the body, can also lead to cramp.

c causes

orm anti-bodies to certain proteins, they will
l' into complexes which act as an inflammatory
ummoning chemicals from your immune system
 the problem elements away. Some people are
 to items in their diet, such as milk proteins or
rotein. Some researchers think that small holes ·
 in the gut lining which allow these proteins
 into body tissues.

 allergy is not a common cause of arthritis, but it
that some people 'do better' if they avoid certain
 is likely that there is an indirect effect of eating
ch of one type of food and not enough of another,
 on making new cartilage, bone or immune cells.
 people are 'allergic' to certain of their own body
hich have an unusual ability to make a complex
eir anti-bodies. This is called auto-immunity, and
toid arthritis is of this type. Blood tests are carried
iscover rheumatoid factors (special anti-bodies)
onfirm the name of the condition. It must be said
se factors are not found in many cases of arthritis,
ne people even have the factors but don't show
, so the picture isn't entirely clear. Ankylosing
litis sufferers generally have an immunoglobulin
 in excess, and this is thought to be hereditary.

Joints

Joints consist of two bones moving against each other.
The end of each bone is covered with cartilage, which is
made of protein and starch very firmly bound together.
Cartilage has no blood vessels or immune system of its
own and is replaced extremely slowly by cells called
chondrocytes. It derives its nutrients and immune cells
from fluid produced by the synovial membrane, which
wraps around the joint.

Deficiency in synovial fluid (sometimes caused by
inflammation) causes stiffness and pain as well as
destruction of cartilage. Production of synovial fluid is
increased by exercise such as walking, skipping, running
and hopping which causes the bone ends to impact
against each other. Muscles surround each joint like layers
of well-organised bandages, with extra strong tendons
attaching them to the underlying bones.

Arthritis and rheumatism explained

What is arthritis?

Arthritis is inflammation of a joint resulting from injury
or infection. It has several features:

- pain
- redness
- heat

- swelling
- immune activity
- destruction
- distortion.

Pain
Pain warns us that something is wrong. The body reacts to pain by tightening the muscles protectively around the joint. As a result movement becomes spasmodic which leads to further pain.

Redness
Redness is caused by extra blood flow in dilated capillaries, to deliver immune factors and dilute irritants.

Heat
Heat is generated by activity of immune cells and dilated blood vessels with extra blood flow.

Swelling
Swelling occurs when fluid, with immune cells, leaks from blood vessels into the surrounding area, causing stiffness in the joint.

Immune activity
The lymph system provides immune cells, which dispose of debris and lymph channels allow it to be cleared away with the extra fluid.

Destruction
 In the process of inflammation ca be destroyed, and acute pain occur grind against each other.

Distortion
Sometimes the whole process of m cartilage becomes so disturbed tha they are not needed and cause dist making the smooth functioning of

Causes of arthritis

There are many different factors w Often several occur together, for e oestrogen levels, heavy manual wo make natural wear and tear worse. very effective in these 'multi-facto of the complexity of herbal consti causative factors in arthritis and r

- allergy
- infection
- crystal deposits
- wear and tear
- poor circulation
- diet
- hormones.

Allerg
If you 'conge agent, to clea allergi wheat develo throug

Foo is clea foods. too m perhap

Som cells, v with th rheum out to which that th and so arthriti spondy (hla27

Infections

Bacterial and viral infections can trigger inflammation in
the joints and muscles, as immune complexes escape into
surrounding tissues from the blood stream. Every one
remembers the awful aching which accompanies 'flu, but
usually our body overcomes the infection and symptoms
subside. In some forms of infection the inflammation
becomes chronic, unfortunately no one really knows why.
It must depend on the state of the immune system, the
tissues, circulation, nutrition and a whole load of other
factors which we might look at in the wholistic way of
researching disease.

Crystalline disorders

Acids (such as uric acid) are a normal by-product of
digestion, especially of proteins. Sometimes the body fails
to eliminate enough and they build up in the blood
stream where they damage the lining to blood vessels and
escape into surrounding tissue. They may complex with
immune proteins and, where they accumulate in a joint,
they cause inflammation, swelling and acute pain. Gout is
one of the crystalline arthritis conditions.

Wear and tear

In some people the cartilage becomes worn away as they
get older and is not replaced. Exposed bone ends grind on
each other causing pain and damage.The bone may

become deformed as a result of uneven wear and replacement, causing stiffness and distortion of the joint. This makes movement and grip very difficult. Osteoarthritis is this sort, it is often known as a 'cold arthritis' as little inflammation is involved, whereas the rheumatoid type is a 'hot arthritis' in which heat and swelling occur. People often have both, or one after the other, just to complicate the picture!

Injury

Injury doesn't just mean the result of a fall or being hit. It can be caused by excessive weight carrying, for example in obesity, or in professions where loads are carried frequently, or in daily shopping where bags are carried for some distance. Injury can also be caused by over-use, such as in professional dancers, or in excessive high-impact sport such as jogging or squash. We might call all these examples of repetitive strain injury, though nowadays the term is usually taken to mean a muscle or tendon problem.

Poor circulation

There are several causes of poor circulation, such as narrowed arteries, vascular tension or anaemia. This leads to insufficient nutrients and oxygen being delivered to joints and muscle, and poor clearance of metabolic waste products. Lymph drainage should be considered in this category, as it is vital for resolving inflammation.

Muscular exercise increases lymph and blood flow by squeezing the channels, as does massage.

Dietary causes

Gout used to be associated with high purine foods and drinks such as port wine and red meat, or with oxalic acid sources such as Indian Spinach and Rhubarb. Despite avoiding these, some people still suffer attacks of gout and it is now thought that they have a problem in getting rid of certain acids from the body. High cholesterol levels may also play a role in formation of acid complexes which cannot be eliminated by the kidney.

Deficiencies of vitamins (which take part in the repair process), minerals and proteins may all play a part in the development of arthritis. Essential fatty acids (contained in vegetable, fish and seed oils) are important for the production of anti-inflammatory agents in the body. Deficiencies in these may play a significant role in chronic joint inflammation.

It is said that refined carbohydrates such as white flour and sugar create acid conditions in the body which favour the development of crystalline arthritis, but a low PH is usually overcome in the intestine. It may be what they lack rather than what they contribute to the blood, or our excessive reliance on them which causes a problem.

Hormonal causes

Most people have heard of the connection between female hormones and osteoporosis. Oestrogen controls the deposition of calcium in bones, essential for growth of babies in the womb. It is essential for women to replace the calcium which is lost to their babies, as well as other nutrients. When levels fall after menopause, unless steps are taken to support oestrogen levels, osteoporosis may develop, leading to spinal deformity and fractures.

Men also suffer from osteoporosis by some unexplained hormonal factor. What is not clear, is why more women suffer from inflammatory arthritis than men. This tendency often develops in menopause. Several factors, including diet, lifestyle and hormones must play a part.

What is rheumatism?

Most people describe rheumatism as a chronic (long lasting) ache in the muscles. It isn't a very well defined condition and nowadays people tend to use the term arthritis instead.

Causes of rheumatism

- cold temperatures
- poor circulation
- lack of exercise

- inflammation
- over-use.

Sufferes will often say that it comes on in rainy weather. There may be some truth in this, as rain is often accompanied by a sudden lowering in temperature, the surface of the skin cools rapidly and blood supply to the muscles is suddenly lowered, causing aching.

In the British climate damp weather is very pervasive, and clothes soak up water imperceptibly, increasing the cooling effect on skin. We know about the dangers of 'wind chill', when our body temperature falls uncomfortably although the thermometer isn't registering very low figures. Damp clothes have a similar effect. It is clear that efficient circulation and warm, dry climates (and clothing!) play a role in maintaining healthy muscles. It should not go without saying that exercise is the main way to improve circulation to muscles.

When you exercise
The blood vessels serving your muscles and skin dilate, helping to remove metabolic deposits and cool you down.

In cold, damp air
Blood vessels constrict in skin and muscles to conserve heat, metabolic waste (such as lactic acid) isn't cleared and aching results.

2

What conventional medicine can offer

If you visit your doctor with symptoms of arthritis, he or she may arrange x-rays to confirm the extent of the disease, and offer you a range of medicines to relieve pain and inflammation. This will include:

- non-steroidal anti-inflammatories
- pain-relievers
- steroids
- gold injections
- HRT for women.

How conventional medicines work

NSAIDs

NSAIDs (short for non-steroidal anti-inflammatory drugs) include:

- aspirin
- indomethacin
- ibuprofen
- mefenemic acid
- diclofenac (Voltarol).

Some of these are also analgesic (pain relieving) in other ways.

They prevent the production of chemicals which are released by blood cells during the process of inflammation. The most well-known are a series of messenger chemicals called prostaglandins. These are made from essential fatty acids which we get from our food (more about these later). Some prostaglandins increase the inflammation process, but others work to prevent inflammation. Herbalists are very interested in the latter sort as they form part of the 'preventive medicine cabinet' which could help to reduce the number of people suffering from arthritis.

Prostaglandins rely on an enzyme called cyclo-oxygenase for their production, and they are made all over the body for different roles – making mucin to protect the stomach lining from acid, setting temperature, dilating bronchi and kidney blood vessels. Drugs such as the NSAIDs mentioned above, which prevent prostaglandins being produced, may have other effects which are desirable such as reducing a fever. However they may also have unwanted side-effects such as eroding the stomach lining, causing asthma or water retention. Aspirin reduces blood clotting, which may be a good thing if you have an increased tendency to clotting or narrowed arteries, where clots might cause a blockage (thrombosis). Aspirin is also a general analgesic, as it acts on nerve endings to reduce pain sensitivity, but this action can also produce whistling (tinnitus) in the ears and is associated with stomach ulcer formation.

Pain-relievers

Codeine-like drugs such as co-dydramol (Distalgesic), co-proxamol and their stronger relative, morphine, act on the brain to reduce sensitivity to pain. They also reduce muscle movement, causing digestive problems such as constipation, nausea, drowsiness and liver damage in large quantities.

Paracetomol works on prostaglandins, but in the brain rather than in the body tissue, so it has far fewer side-effects but is noted for causing permanent liver damage in large doses.

Steroids

This is a group of chemicals based on the natural hormones we produce in our adrenal glands called gluco-corticoids (for sugar and fat metabolism, building and repair) and mineralo-corticoids (for mineral and water balance). Most steroids have both types of activity; prednisolone, betamethasone, dexamethasone and hydro-cortisone all have more gluco-corticoid than other actions.

Steroid drugs work by preventing enzymes from breaking down cells and by preventing the production of inflammatory chemicals such as prostaglandins. Natural steroids, produced in the body, have a large number of functions, mainly to do with 'prioritising' the use of nutrients from digestion. This includes making protein structures such as muscle, skin and immune cells, storing sugars and fats as well as balancing minerals such as sodium and potassium. Adrenal hormones also affect emotional reactions as part of the human response to attack system.

Needless to say, any drug which affects these fundamental processes by mimicking or blocking adrenal hormones will have wide-ranging effects in the body. Thinning skin and blood vessel walls, re-directing fat, creating appetite, retaining water, reducing immune responses and increasing aggression are known side-effects of using steroids. A commonly observed effect of long-term steroid use is a lift in mood, often not noticed until lower doses are tried and depression sets in.

Gold therapy

This consists of specially formulated gold, injected directly into the joint. No one knows how it works, it is thought to suppress fundamental immune reactions. There is no information about how the therapy originated, and little about its success rate. It is very toxic to kidneys and bone marrow and is most often used as a one-off injection treatment.

The treatments mentioned above, together with HRT for women, form the current conventional approach to arthritis and rheumatism. Large doses of single chemicals usually have quick effects but troublesome side-effects set in after a short while. For many sufferers it is a question of juggling the need to control debilitating pain with the discomfort and danger to health of some side-effects.

~ 3 ~

Using herbs to treat Arthritis and Rheumatism

When herbalists make up a prescription for a patient with arthritis, they take into account all the factors which contribute to the condition of the joints, and try to improve all the systems which affect the joints. This is called a wholistic approach, and it is the main difference between conventional treatment and herbal treatment. In addition to prescribing herbal medicine herbalists would want a patient to include exercises and dietary changes in a strategy to create muscle and joint health.

Aims of herbal treatment

The main aims of herbal treatment are to:
- improve circulation and lymph flow
- reduce inflammation
- relieve swelling and pain
- improve nutrient absorption
- relax muscles
- reduce nervous tension
- balance hormones and immune system.

The patient is prescribed herbs which are intended to improve blood and lymph circulation, halt the inflammatory process, take away excess fluid (via lymph and kidneys), help absorption of essential nutrients using digestive stimulants, relax muscles and relieve pain.

In addition to treating all the factors directly involved in the development of arthritis, we might treat ailments which are indirectly involved, for example nervous tension, which may increase muscular tension and pain. Chronic pain is very stressful and often results in mild depression, so we might prescribe nervine relaxants to relieve this.

The immune system plays a leading role in arthritis, and there are several herbs with unique actions on the immune system, making it more efficient in defeating infections or less reactive to allergens. These are what we call balancing actions and we use them in other body systems.

We can use herbs to balance the female hormone system, so that women don't suffer worse symptoms in the last two weeks of their menstrual cycle when water retention is increased and emotions are more variable. Many herbs and foods contain phyto-oestrogens (plant hormones), which help to maintain bone and joint health in menopause.

Individual compound remedies

We might be concerned to offset some of the side-effects

of conventional medication, so we could provide herbs which protect and restore the lining of the stomach. If a patient has been taking medicines which damage the liver, we would add liver tonics. If anaemia results from disease or medication, we would use iron-rich herbs, and if the blood vessel walls have become fragile, we will add herbs which contain bio-flavonoids to strengthen the blood vessel walls. Last but not least, if pain has interrupted sleep patterns, there are herbs which induce sleep and improve its quality.

This sounds complicated, but by careful choosing, you can make up a compound remedy which suits you. You may need to experiment a little but none of the herbs mentioned in this book are dangerous. Sample recipes are presented later with the case histories, and there is a list of sources at the end of the book if you need more help.

Combining herbs with orthodox medication

Some drugs are altered by liver enzymes, so that they enter the main blood circulation in a different form. Some herbs (especially bitters) stimulate the liver cells to work harder, or cause more liver cells to be active, and this can affect other drugs because the liver removes them from circulation before they have had a chance to do their work. Digoxin is one of these and it is also a drug with a 'narrow therapeutic window'. This means that the difference between an insufficient, a beneficial and a harmful dose is very small, so that small changes in the amount getting through to the bloodstream may result in the drug not working as it should. Two other drugs like this are Cyclosporin, used to prevent transplant rejection, and Phenytoin, an anti-epileptic. It is very important to check with a qualified herbalist and let your doctor know if you are adding herbal medicine to medication you are currently using.

Safe combining

There are many herbs which can be taken safely with other medicines, so don't feel deterred from trying, but do seek professional advice. Herbs can be used to offset the side-effects of necessary medication, like indigestion or nausea. They may enable you to take less of a remedy which you need, but which has troublesome side-effects. The important thing is how you feel, and that you don't endanger your health. It may be simple to ask your doctor to monitor blood levels of drugs and adjust the dose if necessary.

It would not be wise to embark on herbal medicine without medical supervision if you are on anti-psychotic medication as you may not be aware that your mental condition has deteriorated when your current medication ceases to work. You may have strong feelings about the disadvantages of your drugs, but may not realise how your behaviour is changing and affecting others badly. It is possible to have herbal medicine for other complaints while on medication for psychosis, but you must consult your doctor first and allow yourself to be monitored. If you are on chemotherapy for cancer, it would be better to wait until your treatment has finished before taking herbal medicine, unless you are looking for help with troublesome side effects such as nausea or diarrhoea. Several herbs can help here without reducing the effectiveness of your anti-cancer drugs.

Drugs to be careful with

- Digoxin
- Phenytoin
- anti-psychotics
- immune suppressants
- anti-cancer drugs.

Conditions to be careful with

- pregnancy
- epilepsy
- schizophrenia, psychosis
- organ transplants
- allergies.

Sometimes over the counter herbal medicines are labelled with contra-indications. This is required by law in Germany. It means, for example, that you will be told if you shouldn't take the medicine if you are pregnant, taking another specific medication, have an allergy or a certain medical condition. This will become more common throughout Europe in the near future.

How herbs work

Herbs contain small quantities of chemicals, compared to modern pharmaceutical products which extract or synthesise one chemical in much larger amounts. Valerian, for example, appears to improve the quality of your sleep as well as helping you to doze off and doesn't cause a sluggish feeling in the morning, unlike many pharmaceutical products. This is because the chemicals it contains are in very small amounts and don't last long in the body. This lower level of activity may be disappointing if you want to be 'knocked out', but using herbs like Valerian as part of a plan to restore sleep patterns can be an effective alternative to stronger single chemicals like the well-known sedative valium (derived originally from valerian).

Synergy of herbal chemicals

Most herbs contain a large number of active constituents which work together to create one or more effects. The more we find out about herbs, the more we realise that each constituent is a valued part of the whole, negative effects balanced by positive ones. A good example follows.

Recently, much has been made of a research trial which showed that a St John's Wort preparation made liver enzymes more active, which reduced the effect of other drugs taken at the same time because they were metabolised before reaching their target. The St John's Wort preparation used was standardised to contain a larger amount of one constituent – hypericin – than all the others. Not only has hypericin failed to show anti-depressant activity on its own in repeated trials, but another ingredient – hyperforin – has been shown to counterbalance hypericin in its effect on liver enzymes. Many other research trials on St John's Wort have shown no adverse effect on other drugs and doctors in Germany continue to prescribe it as a favoured anti-depressant.

Similar bad publicity surrounds Liquorice, where glycyrrhizin is thought to raise blood pressure, but in fact dozens of other constituents act to lower it, in particular by diuresis (elimination of water). There are many more examples of this sort of balanced action. Where two or more constituents act together to create the same effect this is known as synergy. These are particular features of herbal medicine which enable it to support the wholistic approach very well.

How long herbs take to work

Although some herbs act swiftly, like the relaxant Valerian, herbal remedies generally act slowly and their effect is cumulative. They gently rebalance physiological processes, as though switch after switch is thrown until the full effect is achieved. This can take weeks, sometimes months, but it is worth waiting for as the risk of side-effects is very low, due to the tiny amounts of chemicals involved.

How herbal remedies get to their target

Herbal compounds need to be absorbed across the wall of the digestive tract, so first they have to be released from their structures (stem, root, leaf, flower or berry etc). Hot water and alcohol do some of this job for us, so that teas and tinctures are more easily absorbed than tablets and capsules, which need to be broken down physically before the active chemicals are separated from the inert matter to which they are attached. All food and medicine passes through the liver (in the blood circulation) before it finally enters the body tissues, where it is used.

Sometimes chemical compounds need help in crossing through the wall of the digestive tract into the blood stream. Carrier chemicals can be attached to compounds and ferry them through channels in the gut lining. Hydrochloride is frequently found to be part of conventional drug names as it has this function.

Herbal compounds often have an advantage over synthesised chemicals in this respect as, they have naturally occurring carrier chemicals already attached to them. This is what is meant by affinity. Herbs are said to have a greater affinity for the human body, like spare parts dedicated to a particular engine made by the same manufacturer.

The advantages of using whole plant preparation

Herbalists insist on using whole, unaltered products to guarantee the sort of benefits we claim for them. We believe that plants would only have gained a historical reputation for certain effects if their constituents were robust enough to maintain the same effect wherever they were grown or whatever minor differences there might be between local plant populations. If only one variety in one particular year made someone feel better its reputation would not have stood the test of time.

Standardisation

The current trend, based on scientific research, is to standardise the process of growing, harvesting and storing herbs, so that their use is sustainable and patients get the best value from them. Medical herbalists also recommend using whole, unaltered preparations, as nature presented them, so that each constituent is represented in its natural amounts. This is the type of preparation on which traditional knowledge is based. It is also useful to remember that patients vary much more than plants do!

Many herbs show a greater affinity for the human body than do synthetic medicines. This is because they have compounds and molecules attached which make them more easily absorbed into body cells and tissues, these are often in the 'sugar ' family, some are known as glycosides. These and their relatives, monosaccharides, are attracting a lot of interest in the modern research world. These carrier chemicals enable herbal compounds to enter target cells more easily, and may explain how herbs can have an effect, even at quite low doses.

One of the great advantages of herbal medicine is that there are so many different plants with similar actions, but different combinations of constituents. You can change from one to the other to avoid becoming tolerant or developing sensitivities. For example there are many anti-inflammatory herbs, each with its own supplementary action, including hormonal, diuretic, anti-spasmodic and relaxing effects. Herbs may act on several different aspects of a condition at the same time, like Garlic which provides help for our circulation on several levels. As an antibiotic, it repairs the damage caused by wear and tear on the insides of our blood vessels. As a digestive stimulant it helps the absorption of sugars and fats from the bloodstream. As a circulatory tonic it reduces the stickiness of platelets, dilates the capillaries, causes mild sweating and increases kidney activity, so it helps to protect against strokes and lowers blood pressure slightly.

Herbal applications

Herbal remedies include conventional applications such as:

- anti-inflammatories
- diuretics (often called kidney tonics by older herbalists)
- pain relievers
- iron tonics.

You could obtain all these from your doctor.

You can also find herbs whose actions are not found in conventional drug descriptions. Mostly this is because of their complexity, which is best reflected in the older names for their applications. We can include here:

- cleansing herbs
- relaxants
- circulatory tonics
- rubefacients
- digestive tonics
- tonic bitters
- healing herbs
- hormonal agents.

You would not expect to obtain these from your doctor.

Anti-inflammatories

This is the most important group of herbs for people with disorders such as arthritis, where inflammation causes so much pain and damage if unchecked. They work by intervening in the inflammatory process at different levels. Some act by reducing the number of immune cells produced in response to injury, for example Chamomile reduces mast cells which are part of the swelling process. Some herbs stabilise cell membranes so they don't break down or allow excess secretion. This may be done by inhibiting chemicals such as bradykinin, serotonin and histamine, which also make small blood vessels leak fluid. It is thought that mucus membrane tonics such as Elderflower work in this way.

Other herbs, like Nettles, are known to inhibit chemicals such as leukotrienes and lymphokines, which increase the production of immune cells. Many cleansing and circulatory tonic herbs are said to be anti-inflammatory because they help to carry away the products of inflammation. Of course, it is common to find herbs which have several or all of these actions at once.

Cleansing herbs

There is another group of herbs whose actions are not so well understood, but they are effective in arthritic, rheumatic and skin problems. These are the cleansing herbs, sometimes known as depurative, purifying or even (that hideous modern word) detoxifying. This group includes traditional favourites such as Dandelion and Burdock, Sarsaparilla, Cleavers and Yellow Dock. Diuretics and liver tonics are considered to be cleansing agents.

Cleansing herbs stimulate activity and increase elimination from organs such as liver, kidneys, bowels, skin and lymph system, so they may be referred to as digestive, hepatic or lymphatic eliminatives. This may help to reduce acid crystals remaining in joints and remove fatty wastes from glands below the skin, or help the liver remove toxins as well as clearing the bowel of bacterial or fungal overload. They are also known as eliminative, alterative, and depurative and are thought to aid clearance of irritating inflammatory or toxic chemicals from tissues. This is particularly important in clearing acid wastes from joints in gouty types of arthritis and in removing metabolic waste from muscles (such as lactic acid).

Many herbs have secondary cleansing actions, especially those which have a bitter tonic action on the liver.

Generally the body does these things very well without help and it's likely that people with no health problems don't need 'detoxifying' (provided they eat a healthy diet), but it would do no harm in the case of an ailment such as acne or arthritis to try the old-fashioned cleansing approach first. Details on how to make herbal teas are given on page 93.

Diuretics (included in cleansing in the Directory of Useful Herbs)

These increase the elimination of water (and solutes) via the kidneys. There are three main types:

1 Osmotic diuretics (such as sugars) contain compounds which attract water to them and carry it out of the body.

2 Metabolic stimulants (such as caffeine) increase the rate at which water is circulated and eliminated.

3 Electrolytic compounds (such as loop diuretics) change the balance of sodium and potassium entering and leaving cells in the kidneys, resulting in more urination.

Iron tonics

These provide iron in a concentrated form, which can make up depleted stores in the body. Iron is found in foods in two forms: haem and non haem iron. Haem iron is found in meat and animal products, and is already metabolised into an easily absorbable form. Non-haem iron is found in plant foods and requires an extra metabolic step to convert it into an absorbable. Both forms are absorbed better when accompanied by vitamin C, so plant sources of iron which contain this vitamin can be a viable alternative to meat.

Pain relievers

Pain relievers are also known as analgesics and anodynes.

There are three different types of analgesic, effective in muscle and joint pain.

1 Central acting analgesics stop the brain from receiving

messages from the periphery. Passionflower, Lettuce leaf, Poppy and St John's Wort work in this way.

2 Herbs such as Silver Birch and Wintergreen have a local action and are applied topically.

3 Anti-inflammatories, like the ones described above, and muscle relaxants such as Cramp Bark and Wild Yam, act on the processes which cause pain.

4 Herbal pain relief is a little slower than conventional medicine.

It can sometimes take two to three days for a full effect to build up, but it's well worth waiting for as it seems to last longer and there are no associated problems.

Relaxants

Unlike sedatives which reduce brain activity to below normal functioning level, herbal relaxants relieve tension and restore nervous activity to a normal level. This can improve concentration rather than impairing it, so it is a good example of a balancing action for which herbs are well known. These herbs work in two ways.

1 Nervine relaxants act centrally, by reducing the brain's sensitivity to nerve messages from the periphery (skin, joints, muscles etc).

2 Muscle relaxants act peripherally (on nerve centres in the spinal cord, or on nerve endings in the skin),

reducing the number of messages sent from the periphery to the brain.

Many herbs have both central and peripheral actions.

Circulatory tonics

These herbs increase the flow of blood to skin and muscles by local irritation and when taken internally, they cause sweating (diaphoresis) which brings with it dilation of blood vessels in the skin. They may dilate blood vessel walls by nerve action – these are the peripheral circulatory tonics. Some circulatory tonics act on the heart to improve performance. These are called centrally acting agents and are mostly used by individuals with specific circulatory problems, and not as part of a general arthritis or rheumatism treatment.

Rubefacient essential oils

These are applied to the skin, where they irritate nerve endings in capillaries and cause redness, which is a sign of greater blood flow through dilated vessels. This in turn causes better perfusion of joints and muscles, relieving them of metabolic wastes which may be causing pain. Very strong rubefacients, such as chilli, have a counter-irritant action, that is the heat overwhelms pain receptors so that fewer messages are sent back to the brain about any sort of pain. Aromatic essential oils are almost all rubefacient in a gentle way, so are recommended for regular use in massage for arthritis and rheumatism.

Digestive tonics

These work by stimulating digestive secretions in the mouth, stomach, pancreas and liver. Bitters are noted for their action on the liver, increasing bile flow which emulsifies fats and transports excess from the bloodstream. Pungent herbs (hot spices) irritate linings which respond by increased secretion of digestive enzymes. These break down starch, fat and protein as well as transporting essential vitamins and minerals across the gut wall into the blood circulation. Aromatic herbs stimulate the digestive tract in a similar way, though more gently, and they reduce bacterial fermentation which causes wind and colic. They usually also contain bitters. The aromatic bitters are well known as part of the British cookery tradition, especially in association with meat dishes. Famous examples are sage with pork and rosemary or mint with lamb.

Tonic bitters

Bitter remedies are unique to herbal medicine. They were the mainstay of herbal manufacturers years ago. 'Tonic bitters' were sold in every pharmacy, and 'tonic stout' was prescribed for elderly patients as well as breastfeeding mums by doctors on the NHS until the early 1970s. Many of the famous herbal tonics are still based on bitters, nearly every country has a national favourite. The French drink gentian wine, Swedes export their bitters, the British put theirs in stouts and beers, Italians prefer vermouth, Mexicans use angostura (which gave us pink gin).

How do bitters work?

Bitter taste buds are located at the back of your tongue. They are designed to detect poisons and trigger a gag reflex, so you spit out food which is bad for you. Humans can overcome the bitter revulsion reflex by three methods: telling ourselves it's good for us, adding nice flavours or adding alcohol! The body however, still working to the primeval instruction handbook, initiates a process to rid the body of unwanted chemicals. The liver produces more enzymes and bile in response to messages sent to the brain from the taste-buds. Saliva flows abundantly to cleanse the mouth, activity in the stomach and pancreas increases, resulting in better absorption of nutrients and elimination of toxins. Pre-dinner drinks are good for you after all!

A recent hospital trial showed that patients who received nasty tasting medicine recovered more quickly than those whose medicine tasted bland. The effect was thought to be psychological, patients felt better because they thought their horrible medicine was more effective. Herbalists think that the bitter effect might have played a tonic role in this experiment.

Healing herbs

Some herbs, such as marigold, heal wounds by increasing growth of new blood vessels and forming scar tissue. These act locally, by application to the skin. The type of healing required in arthritis and rheumatism is more like rebuilding – in the old sense of the word heal, to make whole. Most of this action comes from plant foods taken medicinally, which will be described in the next chapter. One herb, comfrey, stands out for having a traditional use in the relief of arthritis and restoring healthy joints.

Hormonal agents

Some herbs provide chemicals which behave like hormones in the human body. The most well known are phyto-oestrogens which have a number of actions. Some occupy sites that human hormones might take up and so block an action, giving a protective effect against cancers which 'feed' on hormones such as oestrogen. Other herbs appear to reduce fibroid growth and excessive menstrual bleeding by an unknown hormonal action. These are often referred to as 'astringents' by herbalists.

Some herbs contain oestrogen-like compounds which appear to relieve menopausal problems such as hot flushes and diminished bone density. We can select the right sort of hormonal herb for our wholistic purpose. For example black cohosh relieves hot flushes and protects against breast-cell overgrowth, so is ideal for women who have had breast cancer or have an increased risk factor for it. This herb also increases circulation and is mildly anti-inflammatory, so for menopausal women with arthritis it seems ideal. Some herbs, such as liquorice, act on the adrenal gland and so help to restore the function of this organ after prolonged use of steroids.

There are a number of herbs which have a hormonal action which may help to achieve overall health in women who suffer worse muscle and joint pain during the menopause. The hormonal effects of herbs are the subject of a great deal of research which will, we hope, help to explain their traditional use in helping problems of hormone imbalance.

Some worries have been expressed about using these if a woman has suffered from cancer of the breast, womb, cervix or ovaries, in case the plant hormones could stimulate further tumorous growth. All the evidence of recent research shows that these herbs have a protective effect against cancer and are very safe. It would be wise, however, to avoid taking them during chemotherapy, such as with Tamoxifen, as we don't yet know whether they would occupy sites which anti-cancer drugs are designed to reach, so blocking the effect of treatment. Some trials have shown safety in this regard, but there aren't enough to be conclusive. It would be better to use nervine herbs (see relaxants) to help control symptoms such as hot flushes during treatment.

Gradual change

It is clear that herbs are similar in action to modern chemical drugs (which are after all mostly designed on herbal models), but plants are complex and the chemicals they contain are in much smaller quantities, so they are often used differently. Persistence is usually more important than quantity – a little every day will slowly bring about change in physiological conditions. The combined advantages of synergy, low dosage, multilevel action, high affinity and low incidence of side effects have ensured that they will continue to be used as well as modern drugs in treatment of all kinds of disease.

4

Directory of useful herbs

You will need to use a number of strategies to relieve arthritis and rheumatism and prevent further deterioration. Preventive approaches are covered in the chapter on eating and exercising for healthy muscles, bones and joints. You can use the information in this section to select the right herbs. The case histories in Chapter 7 guide you in building classic recipes, or tailoring one to your own individual needs.

Herbs are usually categorised by their actions, and each herb will have some primary and some secondary actions. In some the actions are of equal importance. Each herb is only listed once for convenience, according to its main action. To treat arthritis and rheumatism we use anti-inflammatories, cleansers, iron tonics, pain relievers, relaxing herbs, circulatory tonics, healing herbs, rubefacients, bitters and digestive tonics and hormonal agents. When you read the case histories presented later you will see how this directory can be used to pick herbs from the various categories to suit you.

ANTI-INFLAMMATORY HERBS

Black cohosh	Ginger	Poplar
Celery seed	Guaiac	Willowbark
Devil's claw	Liquorice	
Feverfew	Meadowsweet	

Black cohosh

Latin name	Cimicifuga racemosa
Origin	America
Part used	Rhizome
Dose	1 teaspoon per cup, 1-2 cups per day. Tincture 2ml, 1-2 times daily
Constituents	Bitter glycosides, isoflavones, isoferulic acid, volatile oil tannins, salicylates, resins
Primary actions	Hormonal agent Anti-inflammatory
Secondary actions	Relaxant
How it works	Isoflavones attach to oestrogen receptors in the body and help to balance the hormone system. They also cause blood vessels and mind to relax, which helps to lower blood pressure. Salicylates act on prostaglandins to reduce inflammation and it is thought that isoferulic acid has a similar action; it also has a possible ovarian action. The glycosides are bitter and provide a tonic digestive effect. Its resins and tannins act astringently on the gut wall to prevent diarrhoea and it is thought there may be a similar action on the wall of

	the womb, as it has some reputation for reducing proliferative growth (fibroids etc).
Caution	This herb is not to be used in pregnancy, where it may affect hormonal support of the foetus. High doses can produce low blood pressure and a sensation of vertigo. Keep to the recommended dose, which is entirely safe.
Growing guide	Once a popular Victorian garden plant, Black Cohosh (Cimicifuga) will grow in damp semi-shade. Still available from nurseries as a potted plant.

Celery seed

(see Cleansing herbs page 58)

Devil's claw

Latin name	Harpagophytum procumbens
Origin	Africa
Part used	Tuber
Dose	1 teaspoon per cup, 1-2 cups daily
	Tincture 5ml daily
Constituents	Iridoid glycosides, flavonoids, phenols, quinones, triterpenes, acids
Primary actions	Anti-inflammatory
Secondary actions	Relaxant
How it works	No one has identified which constituent has the most active effect on inflammation. Flavonoids promote blood vessel health and water elimination, phenols are anti-

inflammatory, iridoid glycosides are bitter and known to increase bile secretion, so improve digestion and cleansing via the liver.

Caution   This herb is not to be used in pregnancy as it may stimulate muscles in the uterus. It is being over-collected in the wild, becoming endangered. Better to buy sustainable herbs like others in this chapter and support projects to cultivate devil's claw in Africa.

Growing guide   May only grow in hot desert conditions, no successful cultivation programmes yet.

Feverfew

Latin name   Tanacetum parthenium
Origin   Europe
Part used   Leaf
Dose   1 teaspoon per cup, one cup per day
                       Tincture 2ml, 1-2 times daily
Constituents   Volatile oil, sesquiterpene lactones, bitters
Primary actions   Pain reliever
                       Anti-inflammatory
Secondary actions   Relieves fever
                       Bitter digestive tonic
How it works   The sesquiterpene lactones inhibit the inflammatory chemical, serotonin, prostaglandins which carry pain messages and some of the white blood cells which are over-produced in rheumatoid arthritis. Both the bitters and the volatile oil are tonic to the digestion It is most famous for its effect on

	blood vessels in migraine.
Growing guide	Sow under glass or directly in soil in late spring. Self seeds all over the garden.

Ginger

Latin name	Zingiber officinalis
Origin	Asia
Part used	Rhizome
Dose	$1/3$ teaspoon to a cup, 1-2 cups per day
	Tincture 2ml daily
Constituents	Volatile oil (camphene, eucalyptene), shogaols, gingerols
Primary actions	Circulatory tonic
	Stimulating digestive tonic
Secondary actions	Anti-inflammatory
How it works	The shogaols (produced in drying) and gingerols act on the stomach wall, reducing sensitivity and nausea. They cause dilation of blood vessels, easing flow of blood both to the digestive system and the peripheral areas of the body. They are also known to inhibit prostaglandin synthesis, by this they reduce inflammation.

Guaiac (other name lignum vitae)

Latin name	Guaiacum officinale
Origin	America
Part used	Resin
Dose	3ml tincture 1-3 times daily. (note: resins don't mix easily with water, so alcoholic

	extracts are preferred)
Constituents	Lignans, terpenoids, acids, saponins
Primary actions	Anti-inflammatory
Secondary action	Cleansing herb depurative
How it works	There is no clear account of this herb's anti-inflammatory action. Resins cause the blood vessels to dilate and increase elimination of water. Saponins are noted for their ability to affect the flow of ions in and out of cells, and may be responsible for some of the cleansing (depurative) action.
Caution	The resins are slightly irritant, and may cause digestive disturbance in people with very sensitive digestion.

Liquorice

Latin name	Glycyrrhiza glabra
Origin	Asia, Europe
Part used	Rhizome
Dose	1 teaspoon per cup, 1 –2 cups daily
	Tincture 5ml daily
Constituents	Polysaccharides, saponins, sterols, bitters, flavonoids, coumarins, asparagin, volatile oil
Primary actions	Anti-inflammatory
	Healing herb
	Hormone agent (adrenal)
Secondary actions	Expectorant
	Anti-spasmodic
	Antacid
	Cleansing herb (diuretic)

How it works   Polysaccharides are non-calorific sugars
                    which coat the stomach and reduce acidity.
                    They also increase elimination of water by
                    osmosis (the sugars 'pull' water along with
                    them through the urinary system). Saponins
                    allow cells to release toxins and secretions
                    more easily, which helps expectoration of less
                    viscous fluid in the bronchial tubes. Sterols
                    have a healing and anti-inflammatory effect
                    like hydrocortisone but they don't cause skin
                    thinning or fat storage effects. Flavonoids
                    increase the flow of urine, offsetting the
                    sterols' water retaining effects. Coumarins
                    reduce spasm in the digestive system.

Caution   Must not be used in higher than
                    recommended doses if you suffer from high
                    blood pressure, especially avoiding liquorice
                    confectionery which may be very
                    concentrated.

Meadowsweet

Latin name	Filipendula ulmaria
Origin	Europe
Part used	Leaf
Dose	1 teaspoon per cup 1-3 cups per day
	Tincture 5ml, 1-2 times daily
Constituents	Salicylates, phenols, coumarins, flavonoids, tannins
Primary actions	Anti-ulcerative
	Anti-inflammatory

Secondary actions Relieves fever
How it works   Salicylates inhibit prostaglandins which carry
                     messages about fever, pain and
                     inflammation. Coumarins reduce spasm in
                     digestive muscle. Tannins and phenols
                     inhibit bacteria which are involved in ulcer
                     formation. Flavonoids help to strengthen
                     small blood vessels, improve circulation and
                     reduce internal bleeding. Tannins astringe
                     and heal the gut wall.
Growing guide   Likes damp feet and warm head! By a hedge
                     seems to suit it well. Seed to be started under
                     glass and plants set out in autumn or
                     following spring.

Poplar (other name Quaking Aspen)

Latin name   Populus tremuloides
Origin   America, Europe
Part used   Bark
Dose   1 teaspoon per cup, 1-2 cups per day
                     Tincture 5ml daily
Constituents   Salicylates, essential oil (bisabolol)
                     flavonoids, tannins
Primary actions   Anti-inflammatory
Secondary actions Digestive tonic
How it works   Tannins draw the cells of mucous membranes
                     together, so that they secrete less and are less
                     permeable, this makes them less irritable and
                     inflamed and is part of the healing process.
                     Most barks contain tannins – in small doses

they heal the gut wall, in large doses they prevent absorption of vitamins and minerals for a short while after ingestion. The salicylates are not irritant to the stomach as their active form is made once the herb has passed through the gut. They inhibit inflammatory chemical production.

Caution   Not to be taken by people with aspirin allergy, or with drugs which interact with aspirin, such as phenytoin, as its effectiveness may be reduced. Do not take with other anticoagulants, such as Warfarin or Heparin, as small haemorrhages may occur.

Willowbark

Latin name	Salix alba
Origin	Europe
Part used	Bark
Dose	1 teaspoon per cup, 1-2 cups per day
	Tincture 5ml per day
Constituents	Salicylates, tannins,coumarins, phenols, flavonoids
Primary action	Anti-inflammatory
	Pain reliever
Secondary action	Relieves fever
	Digestive tonic
How it works	Salicylates inhibit prostaglandins which mediate pain, fever and inflammation. Tannins astringe and tone the gut wall, reducing movement and water content of

bowel. Unlike aspirin, which can destroy the lining of the stomach with prolonged use, the salicylates in Willowbark are assembled after the remedy has passed through the digestive tract. They can, like aspirin, break down sticky platelets in the blood, so help to maintain blood flow and reduce the risk of thrombosis.

Caution   Do not take if you suffer from an allergy to aspirin. Not to be taken with drugs which interact with aspirin, such as phenytoin, which could be reduced in effect, or with blood thinning drugs such as Warfarin and Heparin, as small haemorrhages may occur.

CLEANSING HERBS

Those which have traditionally been used in arthritis are included here. Cleansing herbs also include diuretics and liver tonics.

Burdock	Kelp	Sarsaparilla
Celery seed	Nettles	Yellow Dock
Dandelion		

You will often find horsetail and cleavers listed as important cleansing herbs, but their affinity is with other body systems (lungs, urinary and lymph) so they are not discussed in this book.

Burdock

Latin name	Arctium lappa
Origin	Europe
Part used	Leaf, root, sometimes seed
Dose	1 teaspoon of leaf or root, 1-2 times daily
	Tincture 5ml daily
Constituents	Bitters, flavonoids, phenols, sugars (inulin)
Primary actions	Cleansing herb
Secondary actions	Anti-infective
How it works	Flavonoids cause diuresis, bitters are tonic to the liver, phenols are anti-infective.
Caution	Don't start use in the middle of an acute gout attack, as it will increase the passage of uric acid crystals, and may make pain temporarily worse.
Growing guide	Damp soil, especially in hedgerows, or on house-side, sown directly in spring.

Celery Seed

Latin name	Apium graveolens
Origin	Europe
Part used	Seed, sometimes leaf
Dose	1 teaspoon of seed, 1-2 times daily
	Tincture 5ml daily
Constituents	Volatile oil, coumarins, (carminative and relaxant – reduce bacterial fermentation and spasm in the gut) flavonoids, phthalides
Primary action	Cleansing herb
	Anti-inflammatory
Secondary action	Relaxant

	Digestive tonic (carminative)
How it works	Flavonoids cause diuresis, coumarins are carminative and relaxant, phthalides are sedative, volatile oil is antiseptic and diuretic.
Caution	Do not start taking in the middle of an acute gout attack, as uric acid crystal elimination is increased, and this may cause increased pain temporarily. Do not take in pregnancy as the volatile oil may stimulate uterine contractions.
Growing guide	Authorities differ, some recommend chalky soil and warm sun by the sea (sounds good!) others say a marshy inland habitat. Try your luck with fresh seed, sown under glass in early spring and transplant to some trial spots. Don't manure, or the plant won't seed so freely.

Dandelion

Latin name	Taraxacum officinalis
Origin	Europe
Part used	Root and leaf
Dose	1 teaspoon of herb or root 1-3 times daily
	Tincture 5ml 1-2 times daily
Constituents	Bitters, phenols, sugars (inulin), vitamin A, sterols, potassium
Primary action	Cleansing herb
	Digestive tonic (bitter)
Secondary action	Heart tonic
How it works	Bitters stimulate liver activity, phenols are

anti-infective, inulin is a non-calorific sugar which promotes diuresis, potassium return to the body acts as a hypo-tensive, reducing strain on the heart. The root is considered more hepatic, the leaf more diuretic. The two are often combined in tincture.

Growing guide   Grows in any soil, direct sowing in spring.

Kelp (Other name Bladderwrack)

Latin name	Fucus vesiculosus
Origin	Europe
Part used	Thallus (whole plant)
Dose	1 teaspoon to one cup, 1-2 times daily
	Tincture 5ml daily
Constituents	Iodine, bitters, mucilage, minerals, phenols, polysaccharides
Primary action	Cleansing herb
	Anti-obesity agent
Secondary action	Nutritive
	Antibiotic
How it works	Iodine and trace elements stimulate the thyroid if it is lacking in these compounds, so help to increase metabolic rate. Polysaccharides stimulate the immune system. Phenols, sulphur and phosphorous compounds are anti-biotic. Minerals contribute to bone formation. Mucilage soothes digestive tract. Bitters stimulate digestion.
Caution	Must be gathered fresh from the sea, not as

drift which loses effectiveness. Avoid
collecting in areas of possible heavy metal
pollution, ie by nuclear energy stations or
outlets from industrial areas, because Kelp
accumulates these.

Nettles

Latin name	Urtica dioica
Origin	Europe
Part used	Leaf
Dose	1 teaspoon per cup, 1-3 cups per day, or in food
	Tincture, 5ml ,1-2 times daily
Constituents	Histamine, serotonin, acetylcholine, vitamin C (fresh), vitamin A, silica, minerals (including iron) flavones, acids
Primary action	Cleansing herb (diuretic)
	Nutritive
	Anti-inflammatory
Secondary action	Anti-haemorrhagic
How it works	Unknown constituents produce anti-inflammatory action, shown in experiments. Silica and other constituents stop bleeding, flavones promote diuresis, improve circulation, minerals improve bone formation, vitamins promote general health,(see page 126).
Growing guide	Any damp soil will do. Bury sections of underground stem just beneath soil surface

in early spring or autumn. Worth growing for butterflies alone!

Sarsaparilla

Latin name	Smilax officinalis
Origin	America
Part used	Root
Dose	1 teaspoon per cup, 1-2 cups per day
	Tincture 5ml daily
Constituents	Saponins, sterols, minerals, essential oil
Primary action	Cleansing herb
	Anti-inflammatory
Secondary action	Iron and mineral tonic
	Nutritive
How it works	Saponins are known to open channels in cell walls, allowing secretions out or chemicals in. Minerals have a tonic nutritive action. The essential oil gives a pleasant flavour to beers and cordials made from this root.
Growing guide	No information on growing in Britain, no known examples.

Yellow Dock

Latin name	Rumex crispus
Origin	Europe
Part used	Root
Dose	1 teaspoon per cup, 1-2 cups per day
	Tincture 2ml 1-2 times daily
Constituents	Tannins, anthraquinones, oxalates, iron bitters

Primary action	Cleansing herb
	Laxative
Secondary action	Iron tonic
How it works	Anthraquinones are absorbed during digestion into the blood where they are circulated back through the gut wall, irritating and stimulating it. This causes the gut muscles to move more rapidly, hence their laxative effect. Oxalate-rich plants (Sorrel, Rhubarb, Dock) have been traditionally used for digestive cancers. Iron is nutritive and the tannins are astringent – all helpful in restoring the wall of the gut. This is a much gentler remedy than senna, and it doesn't cause griping.
Caution	Those who suffer from gout may find the oxalates make their condition worse.
Growing guide	Any soil, freely sow directly in spring. Seeds itself everywhere.

IRON TONICS

Iron is supplied in plant food as well as meat and these sources will be discussed in Chapter 6. Extra iron intake may be important for arthritis sufferers, as there is often an increased breakdown of red blood cells and these need to be replaced.

PAIN RELIEVERS

This includes a number of well known relaxing herbs, as these help reduce the perception of pain.

Passionflower	Silver Birch	Wild Lettuce
Poppy	St John's wort	Wintergreen

Passionflower

Latin name	Passiflora incarnata
Origin	America
Part used	Leaf
Dose	1 teaspoon per cup, 1-2 cups per day
	Tincture, 2ml 1-2 times daily
Constituents	Alkaloids, saponins, flavonoids
Primary actions	Relaxant (mental and muscular)
Secondary actions	Lowers blood pressure
How it works	Alkaloids act on the brain, reducing sensitivity to pain. Those in passionflower are known to work on nerves in the spinal cord which control the movement of blood vessel and digestive muscle. This produces a relaxing effect which lowers blood pressure. The flavonoids supplement Vitamin C in strengthening blood vessels by being laid down in the structure of the muscle wall. This also tends to reduce inflammatory swelling as it reduces leakage through capillary walls.

Poppy

Latin name	Papaver rhoeas
Origin	Europe
Part used	Flower
Dose	1 teaspoon per cup, 1-2 cups per day. Syrup is usually preferred, though hardly obtainable now. You can get tincture of Californian Poppy (Latin name Escholtzia) which is closely related. To make your own red poppy tincture you need to use the petals straight after picking.
Constituents	Alkaloids, meconic acid, mucilage
Primary actions	Pain reliever
	Anti-spasmodic
Secondary actions	Expectorant
How it works	The alkaloids act on the brain to reduce sensitivity to pain messages. Mucilage soothes the gullet and stomach, by reflex action it soothes the bronchial tubes which assists expectoration.
Growing guide	Sow seed direct in the ground in a sunny, well-drained spot in early spring. Collect and process immediately on flowering.

Silver Birch

Latin name	Betula alba
Origin	Europe
Part used	Leaf, bark, distilled oil
Dose	Mainly used externally to relieve rheumatic pain. The leaves may be taken in tea, 1

	teaspoon per cup, 1-2 cups per day
Constituents	Methylsalicylate, volatile oil, flavonoids
Primary action	Pain reliever
Secondary action	Decongestant
	Cleansing herb (diuretic)
How it works	Methylsalicylate in the volatile oil reduces the sensitivity of nerve endings under the skin, which gives pain relief. It also increases circulation, warming and relaxing the muscles. Resins and flavonoids in the leaf increase water elimination via the kidneys and so cleanse joints of acid wastes.
Growing guide	Professional methods are required to extract the oil from managed copses.

St John's wort

Latin name	Hypericum perforatum
Origin	Europe
Part used	Leaf and flower
Dose	1 teaspoon per cup, 1-2 cups per day
	Tincture, 5ml per day
Constituents	Essential oil, hypericin, hyperforin, flavonoids, tannins
Primary action	Anti-depressant
	Relieves anxiety
Secondary actions	Relaxant
	Local pain relief
How it works	The whole herb produces a calming and uplifting effect, which reduces the perception of pain as well as inhibiting painful processes

such as spasm and inflammation. None of the individual constituents have proved to be effective on their own. The oil, applied topically, is anti-inflammatory and analgesic, useful for neuralgia, shingles and earache.

Caution A recent research trial suggests that St John's Wort may make the liver destroy some drugs, which could be important for medicines whose dose has to be very precise, such as anti-epileptics, immune suppressants and heart rhythm regulators. Unfortunately this research was based on a standardised type of St John's Wort, where extra hypericin had been added. No trials using non-modified St John's Wort have shown such results, but we now advise patients who are taking any of the medicines above to avoid this herb and grapefruit, which has the same effect to a greater degree. It is perfectly safe to use externally with any medication except drugs designed to make your skin more sensitive to the sun (some psoriasis sufferers take these).

Growing guide Easy to sow direct in spring, will tolerate most soils.

Wild lettuce

Latin name	Lactuca virosa
Origin	Europe
Part used	Leaf
Dose	1 teaspoon per cup, 1 cup at night

	Tincture 3ml 1-2 times daily
Constituents	Alkaloids, bitters, flavonoids, coumarins
Primary actions	Relaxant
	Pain reliever
Secondary actions	Cough relieving
	Anti-spasmodic
How it works	The alkaloids act on the brain, reducing sensitivity to pain messages. Coumarins are anti-spasmodic, so all muscles relax (bronchial, digestive, and somatic), and tension and irritability are diminished.
Caution	This herb can be quite sedative, so avoid large doses and don't drink this tea before driving. A good drink for night-time relief of pain, with a reputation for curing nightmares which goes back to ancient times.
Growing guide	Sow direct in spring in a sunny spot, protect from birds and slugs.

Willowbark

(see Anti-inflammatories page 56)

Wintergreen

Latin name	Gaultheria procumbens
Origin	America
Part used	Leaf
Dose	External use, using essential oil or leaves in bath and inhaler
Constituents	Methylsalicylate, volatile oil
Primary actions	Pain reliever

	Circulatory stimulant
Secondary actions	Decongestant
How it works	Methylsalicylates reduce sensitivity of nerve endings under the skin, relieving pain. They also increase circulation in the skin, attracting a greater blood flow through joints and muscles underneath. This in turn helps to clear waste metabolites, which cause pain and swelling. Wintergreen is very effective in relieving muscular pain, but cannot really reach large joints, as they lie too deep below the surface. It is excellent for small joints such as fingers and toes. Much back pain consists of spasmodic muscles protecting sore joints, so wintergreen can help here too, especially when a poultice wrap is applied.
Growing guide	A low growing plant with attractive berries which is often grown in British gardens for ground cover. Available in nurseries, but a very large amount and professional equipment are required for essential oil extraction. Leaves can be pulled and infused in the bath and inhaler.

Note

There are a number of stronger pain relievers, which are not available over the counter but must be obtained through consultation with a professional medical herbalist. These include Jamaica Dogwood, Winter Jasmine, Aconite and some anti-spasmodics which will be mentioned in the section on relaxants.

RELAXANTS

Black cohosh	Lemon balm	Skullcap
Chamomile	Limeflowers	Valerian
Cowslips	Passionflower	Vervein
Cramp bark	St John's wort	Wild yam
Kava-kava		

Black Cohosh
(see Anti-inflammatories page 49)

Chamomile

Latin name	Matricaria recutita (this plant has been renamed several times recently, so you must specify small, cone-headed flowers with single row of petals. This is currently called German chamomile)
Origin	Europe
Part used	Flowers
Dose	1 teaspoon per cup, 1-3 cups per day Tincture 5ml, 1-3 times daily
Constituents	Volatile oil, flavonoids, coumarins, valerianic acid, sesquiterpene bitters, salicylates, tannins
Primary actions	Relaxant Digestive tonic
Secondary actions	Anti-spasmodic

How it works	Chamomile is one of the most complex herbs in common use. It has a little of almost every action shown by plants.The volatile oil acts on the brain to reduce sensitivity as well as being mildly antiseptic and anti-inflammatory when applied topically. Flavonoids are mildly diuretic, coumarins relax visceral muscle by acting on local nerve centres. The volatile oil is carminative(reduces bacterial ferment and wind in the gut).Sesquiterpene bitters stimulate bile production in the liver and there are bitter glycosides which add to this action. Anti-inflammatory salicylates are present in small quantities, tannins astringe and tone the wall of the gut, alleviating diarrhoea.
Growing guide	Annual. Sow seeds each year in pots, window boxes or scatter freely in a sunny position in spring.

Cowslips

Latin name	Primula veris
Origin	Europe
Part used	Flowers
Dose	$1/2$ teaspoon per cup
	Tincture 2ml, 1-3 times daily
Constituents	Saponins, volatile oil, flavonoids, phenols, tannins, glycosides
Primary actions	Relaxing herb
	Anti-spasmodic

Secondary actions	Expectorant
How it works	The saponins are expectorant as they increase the production of thin mucus which relieves bronchial tubes from congestion by thick, sticky mucus. The phenols are mildy antibiotic. The anti-spasmodic effect is mainly due to the flavonoids and the glycosides which are similar to aspirin compounds. The cowslip has a very long traditional use for nervous irritability and headaches as well as paralytic ailments (perhaps these were of the nervous variety?). It can be used for all cases of restlessness, especially if you have a tendency to bronchitis or asthma.
Caution	Being over-collected in the wild, buy only cultivated stock.

Cramp bark

Latin name	Viburnum opulus
Origin	Europe
Part used	Bark
Dose	1 teaspoon per cup, 1-3 cups per day
	Tincture 3ml, 1-3 times daily
Constituents	Viburnine, tannin, valerianic acid, coumarins
Primary actions	Anti-spasmodic
Secondary actions	Relaxant
	Digestive tonic
How it works	Coumarins and other constituents relax muscle by reducing the number of messages

sent to the brain. They affect both digestive muscle and skeletal muscle. Valerianic acid acts on the brain to reduce reception of messages, producing a feeling of relaxation. Viburnine is bitter, so has a tonic effect on digestion. The tannins reduce the free flow of water through the gut wall, so help to alleviate diarrhoea.

Caution	Some people feel drowsy when they take this herb, so wait one hour after drinking for the first time to see what effect it has on you before driving or operating machinery.
Growing guide	Easy to grow shrub, green-white flower heads in early spring, available in most garden centres as snowball bush.

Kava-kava

Latin name	Piper methysticum
Origin	South Sea Islands
Part used	Root
Dose	1 teaspoon per cup, 1-2 cups per day
	Tincture 3ml, 1-2 times daily
Constituents	Pyrones, piperidine alkaloids, glycosides, mucilage
Primary actions	Relaxant
	Anti-depressant
Secondary actions	Anti-spasmodic
	Cleansing herb (diuretic)
How it works	Not much is known about the actions of kava-kava, though research is increasing as it

becomes popular. The pyrones and piperidines act centrally (on the brain) to reduce sensitivity to pain. Applied topically it is rubefacient and numbing. It also has a reputation for relieving fatigue, so in some books it is referred to as a stimulant. It is best to view it like alcohol, relaxing and stimulating at the same time, with some effects of intoxication at high doses.

Growing guide   It is not possible in the British Isles.

Lemon Balm

Latin name	Melissa officinalis
Origin	Europe
Part used	Leaf
Dose	1 teaspoon per cup 1-3 cups per day
	Tincture 4ml, 1-3 times daily
Constituents	Volatile oil, flavonoids, phenols, triterpenes, tannins
Primary actions	Relaxant
	Digestive tonic
Secondary actions	Anti-viral
	Anti-thyroid
How it works	The volatile oil has a central relaxing effect (on the brain) as well as reducing thyroid hormone stimulation of other systems. It also inhibits the growth of viruses such as herpes by giving a sort of repellant protection to the tissues, and possibly penetrating viral coating. The phenols add to this effect and

help to dispel bacteria in the gut. Triterpenes are bitter so they stimulate digestive secretions. Tannins astringe the wall of the gut, alleviating diarrhoea.

Growing guide   You will rarely have to resort to seed, nearly everyone has some Lemon Balm to give away. It seeds itself like mad, tolerates any soil and will grow in pots.

Limeflowers

Latin name	Tilia europaea
Origin	Europe
Part used	Leaf and flower
Dose	1 teaspoon per cup, 1-2 cups per day
	Tincture 4ml, 1-3 times daily
Constituents	Volatile oil, flavonoids, phenols, mucilage, tannins
Primary actions	Relaxant
	Lowers blood pressure
Secondary actions	Increases sweating
	Anti-spasmodic
How it works	The volatile oil reduces the brain's sensitivity to pain messages, mucilage soothes the stomach and gut wall and flavonoids make blood vessels less fragile. Phenols are antiseptic and diaphoretic (increase sweating), which induces dilation of blood vessels. The overall effect is to calm and lower blood pressure. Limeflowers is a particularly nice tasting tea.

Growing guide Too large a tree for the average garden, a most magnificent specimen can be seen at Kew Gardens in London.

Passionflower

(see page 64)

Skullcap

Latin name	Scutellaria laterifolia
Origin	America
Part used	Leaf
Dose	1 teaspoon per cup, 1-2 cups per day
	Tincture 3ml, 1-3 times daily
Constituents	Flavonoids, glycosides, iridoids, volatile oil, tannin
Primary actions	Relaxant
Secondary actions	Anti-spasmodic
	(Possibly) anti- inflammatory
How it works	Little is known about the active constituents of America skullcap as most research is based on a Chinese variant. We rely on the tradition of use for our knowledge of its actions. The anti- inflammatory effect is present in the Chinese variety and it is very likely that both varieties have the same constituents. America skullcap is noted for its central (brain) calming effect, flavonoids stabilise blood vessel walls and contribute to its mooted anti-inflammatory effect, as well as mildly increasing the elimination of water

via the kidneys. It has a long traditional use for neurological diseases such as epilepsy and motor neurone diseases.

Growing guide   Prefers damp soil. Sow under glass and plant out in early summer in a warm, damp spot (pond-side, bog-garden).

Valerian

Latin name	Valeriana officinalis
Origin	Europe
Part used	Root
Dose	1 teaspoon per cup, one cup per night
	Tincture 2-5ml nightly
Constituents	Valerianic acid, alkaloids, glycosides, tannins, choline, flavonoids, valepotriates, iridoids
Primary actions	Relaxant/sedative
Secondary actions	Anti-spasmodic
How it works	Valerianic acid and valepotriates reduce excitability of brain and feelings of anxiety. Best used at night as it is on the borderline between relaxants and sedatives. Flavonoids are mildly diuretic (increase water elimination).
Growing guide	Sow directly in a sunny spot with damp soil in early spring.

Vervein

Latin name	Verbena officinalis
Origin	Europe
Parts used	Leaf, flower

Dose	1 teaspoon per cup, 1-3 cups per day
	Tincture 3ml, 1-3 times daily
Constituents	Glycosides, iridoids, bitters, volatile oil, alkaloids, mucilage
Primary actions	Relaxant
	Bitter digestive tonic
Secondary actions	Anti-depressant
	Anti-viral
How it works	Not all actions are clearly understood. Bitters stimulate liver and digestive secretions, unknown constituents act on the brain to reduce sensitivity to pain and increase feelings of well-being. These are probably found in the volatile oil, which is responsible for the anti-viral effect, acting as a repellant in the tissues of the body. This is known as the constitutional effect which French aromatherapists call the terrain theory. The whole herb has some pain relieving action when applied as a poultice to inflamed joints and muscles.
Growing guide	Sow under glass, plant out in late spring. Vervein is a very delicate looking plant which will seed itself readily in sunny spots.

Wild yam

Latin name	Dioscorea villosa
Origin	America
Part used	Rhizome
Dose	1 teaspoon per cup, 1-2 cups per day

	Tincture 2ml, 1-3 times daily
Constituents	Saponins, sterols, tannins, starch
Primary actions	Muscle relaxant
	Hormonal agent
Secondary actions	Anti-spasmodic
How it works	Sterols and saponins are oestrogenic so have various effects in the hormone system, for example reducing menopausal flushes and vaginal dryness. It appears to relax the digestive system and prevent colic in both men and women, possibly by some anti-inflammatory effect of the saponins on the gut wall.
Growing guide	Not possible in the British Isles.

NOTE

There are several relaxants and anti-spasmodics which are not available over the counter, but can be obtained by consultation with a qualified medical herbalist. These include lobelia (for bronchial spasm and muscle cramps), Belladonna and henbane (used mainly for kidney colic). See page 139 for how to contact medical herbalists.

CIRCULATORY TONICS

| Chilli | Ginger | Mustard |
| Garlic | Horseradish | Prickly Ash |

Chilli (other name Cayenne)

Latin name	Capsicum minimum
Origin	America
Part used	Fruit
Dose	Depends largely on individual tolerance. Start with one tiny pinch of powder, or one drop of tincture in a little warm water, once or twice daily. Work up to a maximum of 1ml, 1-2 times daily
Constituents	Pungent element (capsaicin), flavonoids, steroidal saponins
Primary actions	Circulatory stimulant
	Digestive tonic
	Pain reliever
Secondary actions	Anti-spasmodic
	Rubefacient
	Anti-septic
How it works	The pungent (hot) compound, capsaicin, causes blood vessels to dilate and skin to sweat by irritation. This creates a feeling of warmth and improves blood flow to all parts. It also stimulates digestive secretions from the mouth onwards, so absorption of nutrients is enhanced. Applied to the skin it produces a strong warming effect called rubefacience, which is described on page 84.
Caution	Can cause pain on an ulcerated stomach or gullet, and intense heat in the mouth, traces on fingers can cause irritation if rubbed into eyes, so care must be taken with the dose and

| | with washing hands after massage. |
| *Growing guide* | Greenhouse or sunny window-ledge. Very attractive and great fun! |

Garlic

Latin name	Allium sativum
Origin	Europe
Part used	Bulb
Dose	1-3 cloves per day (cloves are the separable sections of the bulb)
Constituents	Volatile oil (sulphur compounds- allicin, alliin) germanium, minerals, B vitamins, flavonoids
Primary actions	Antibiotic
	Anti-thrombotic
Secondary actions	Dilates blood vessels
	Increases sweating
How it works	The volatile oil and trace element, germanium, cause sweating. This is accompanied by vasodilation, so blood flow through capillaries increases.
	Note You must crush garlic if you are using the fresh cloves, as two compounds allicin and alliin are released and act on each other to produce the antibiotic effect. Powdered garlic has some of garlic's benefits, but not all of them. To do good it must smell good!
Growing guide	Plant cloves in autumn for following year. Garlic prefers a sunny spot and well-drained soil. You can plant it among your roses,

where it will deter aphids.

Ginger

(see Anti-inflammatories)
The pungent (hot) compounds act in the same way as cayenne but in a gentler manner.

Horseradish

Latin name	Armoracia rusticana
Origin	Europe
Part used	Root
Dose	Usually taken as sauce on nut, meat and fish dishes. Very pungent, so small amounts, $1/2$ teaspoon taken in a bland base such as cream or yoghurt.
Constituents	Glucosilinates (mustard oils), vitamins B and C, asparagine, bitter resin
Primary actions	Digestive tonic Circulatory stimulant
Secondary actions	Diuretic
How it works	When eaten the mustard oils in horseradish stimulate digestive secretions and so enhance absorption of nutrients. They also increase circulation by dilating blood vessels and cause sweating. When applied to the skin the infused oil creates heat (is rubefacient) which helps to relax muscles below. Asparagine increases the elimination of water via the kidneys. Best taken as a regular part of the diet.

Caution	Like all members of the brassica family it should not be overused, as the glucosilinates reduce thyroid activity in large doses. Horseradish oil may be too hot for sensitive skins. Can cause pain if stomach is ulcerated.

Mustard

Latin name	Brassica nigra
Origin	Europe
Part used	Seed
Dose	1/2 teaspoon, 1-2 times daily. Usually taken as sauce with food, also applied as infused oil and in foot baths(one dessertspoon to 2 pints water, infused until lukewarm)
Constituents	Glucosilinates (mustard oils), sinapin, fixed oil, mucilage
How it works	The hot mustard oils, taken internally, produce irritation, feeling of warmth and sweating, which is accompanied by blood vessel dilation. Applied to the skin it warms, relaxes muscles and increases blood flow through the joints beneath. Mustard foot baths have been satirised by cartoonists, but are a surprisingly effective way of counteracting mild hypothermia.

Prickly Ash

Latin name	Zanthoxylum Americaum
Origin	America
Part used	Berries

Dose	$1/2$ teaspoon per cup, 1-2 cups per day
	Tincture 2ml, 1-2 times daily
Constituents	Resin, volatile oil, bitters, coumarins,
	alkaloids, tannin
Primary actions	Circulatory stimulant
	Increases sweating
Secondary actions	Digestive tonic
	Anti-spasmodic
How it works	It is not yet known which compounds cause the effects on peripheral circulation. Coumarins relax muscles in the gut and relieve spasm. Bitters increase liver and digestive secretions. Volatile oil and resins create warmth when applied to the skin, so may also be responsible for the internal circulatory effect.

RUBEFACIENT ESSENTIAL OILS

Cedarwood	Pine	Thyme
Juniper	Rosemary	Wintergreen
Lavender		

These are all used topically (in massage or bath) and contain mildly irritating constituents which increase blood flow to the skin, which in turn causes increased perfusion of tissues underneath, such as muscles and joints.

HEALING HERBS

Most healing actions for muscles and joints come from nutrition
– see Chapter 6.

Comfrey

Comfrey

Latin name	Symphytum officinalis
Origin	Europe
Part used	Leaf
Dose	1 teaspoon per cup, 1-3 cups daily
	Tincture 3ml, 1-3 times daily maximum 8 weeks
Constituents	Mucilage, gum, allantoin, consolidine, choline, tannins, phenols, resin, pyrrolizidine alkaloids (trace in leaf) asparagine, rosemarinic acid
Primary actions	Healer
	Anti-haemorrhagic
Secondary actions	Astringent
How it works	Allantoin, consolidine and other constituents stimulate fibroblast, chondroblast and osteoblast activity, so help to repair worn or damaged cartilage, bone and muscle. Its tannins and mucilage reduce internal bleeding by astringency and demulcent actions. The phenols are antiseptic and anti-inflammatory. Comfrey is noted for its ability to relieve inflammatory swelling when applied as oil or as a poultice, but this action

	is not yet explained.
Caution	Although the amount of pyrrolizidine alkaloids in the leaf is extremely small, and toxicity has only been noted at very high levels of use, it is advised not to exceed 3 cups per day and take for no more than 8 weeks at a time. Using root comfrey (which contains more P. A.'s) has been banned in Britain. These alkaloids are known to accumulate in the liver and obstruct its circulation, but there have been no recorded cases of illness or fatality in Britain at these doses over the hundreds of years of traditional use.
Growing guide	A vigorous herb, tolerates any soil and weather. Propagate from root cuttings from a reliable source (to avoid obtaining varieties with more P. A.'s than the one traditionally used).

DIGESTIVE TONICS

Pungent digestive tonics	Aromatic and bitter digestive tonics
Chilli	Lemon balm
Galangal	Rosemary
Ginger	Sage
Horseradish	Thyme

Chilli

(see Circulatory tonics)

Galangal

Latin name	Alpinia officinarum
Origin	Asia
Part used	Rhizome
Dose	$1/2$ teaspoon per cup 1-2 cups per day Tincture 3ml, 1-3 times daily. Also used in cooking, especially Indonesian dishes. Tastes of cloves and ginger
Constituents	Volatile oil, sesquiterpenes, probably acetoxyeugenol
Primary actions	Digestive tonic
Secondary actions	Carminative
How it works	The aromatic and pungent elements of the volatile oil stimulate digestive secretions and the bitter sesquiterpenes increase liver activity. Some varieties contain acetoxyeugenol, which is anti-septic and carminative (dispels wind and colic)it is likely that commercial stocks of galangal contain different varieties.
Growing guide	Not grown in Britain.

Ginger

(see Anti-inflammatories)

Horseradish

(see Circulatory tonics)

Lemon balm

(see Relaxants)

Rosemary

Latin name	Rosemarinus officinalis
Origin	Europe
Part used	Leaf (oil externally)
Dose	1 teaspoon per cup, 1-2 cups per day
	Tincture 3ml, 1-3 times daily
Constituents	Volatile oil, phenols, flavonoids, tannins,
	bitters, resin
Primary actions	Digestive tonic
	Circulatory tonic
Secondary actions	Anti-inflammatory
How it works	The volatile oil contains several compounds which stimulate nerve endings and produce a sense of warmth. They also stimulate the lining of the digestive system, which responds by secreting more digestive juices. The bitters stimulate the liver to produce more bile, so that fatty meat and nut dishes are more easily digested (hence the famous combination of Rosemary and lamb). The phenols are mildly antiseptic, they reduce fermentation in the gut, alleviating wind and colic. The volatile oil components do penetrate brain tissue, where they facilitate nerve message transmission. This action has given rise to the traditional view that Rosemary improves memory. Research trials

using oils of Sage and Rosemary with elderly
residents of nursing homes have shown
reliably to improve mental function.

Sage and Thyme

Contain similar compounds to Rosemary and have the same
tonic effects on digestion, with different secondary actions. Sage
is mainly known for its hormonal effects in menopause and
Thyme is known as an anti-biotic for respiratory complaints such
as asthma.

All these tonic herbs can be used freely in food, details in
Chapter 6.

HORMONAL AGENTS

Black cohosh	Red clover	Sage

Black cohosh

(see Anti-inflammatory herbs)

Red clover

Latin name	Trifolium pratense
Origin	Europe
Part used	Leaf, flower
Dose	1 teaspoon per cup, 1-2 cups per day
	Tincture 5ml daily
Constituents	Isoflavones (oestrogenic), cyanogenic
	glycosides, coumarins, galactomannans,

	flavonoids
Primary actions	Cleanser
	Hormonal agent
Secondary actions	Anti-spasmodic
	Anti-thrombotic
How it works	The isoflavones are taken up by oestrogen receptors in the body, where they appear to have a protective and balancing effect (hot flushes and irritability diminish). They also have a mild diuretic effect, unlike true oestrogens. The herb has a long anti-cancer reputation which is probably based on its hormonal action. The coumarins are anti-spasmodic and mildly anti-coagulant, so help to prevent thrombosis. The cyanogenic compounds are also anti-spasmodic.

Sage

Latin name	Salvia officinalis
Origin	Europe
Part used	Leaf
Dose	1 teaspoon per cup, 1-2 cups per day
	Tincture 3ml, 1-3 times daily
Constituents	Volatile oil, flavonoids, phenols, thujone, tannins, triterpene bitters, saponins(oestrogenic), resin
Primary actions	Hormonal agent
Secondary actions	Anti-fungal (antiseptic)
	Digestive tonic
How it works	Sage oil has a potent anti-fungal, antiseptic

called thujone. Other components of the oil stimulate the lining of the gut to secrete more, so digestion is enhanced. Its bitters increase liver production of bile, so help fatty meat and nut digestion. Phenols reduce bacterial fermentation, so relieve wind associated with rich dishes. The tannins are astringent both in the throat, where they are traditionally used to relieve infections, and in the gut where they reduce excess mucus and bacteria. The oestrogenic compounds account for its ability to reduce hot flushes in menopause and its antibiotic substances are probably responsible for its reputation in curing night sweats associated with infections, including T.B.

Growing guide   Sage, Rosemary and Thyme share a liking for warm, well drained soil.

❧ 5 ❧

Growing and making
your own herbal remedies

You can prepare herbs in a wide variety of ways to bring comfort and relief to arthritic joints and rheumatic muscles.

Types of herbal preparation

Oral remedies are swallowed in measured doses. They include:

- teas
- tinctures
- syrups
- pills.

Topical remedies are applied to the skin and include:

- creams
- oils
- baths
- plasters and poultices.

Oral remedies

Teas

Teas (also called **tisanes**) can be made directly from dried herbs. Leaves and flowers require five minutes steeping in freshly boiled water. Always place a saucer or cover on the cup to keep in valuable aromatic ingredients. This is known as an **infusion**. Roots, barks, seeds and berries need boiling for five minutes in a covered pan. This is called a **decoction**. The usual dose is one rounded teaspoon per cup (about 4g to 165ml). Regular use means one or two cups per day for several weeks. Infusions and decoctions can be drunk cold, and any flavouring can be added after steeping or boiling.

- To make an infusion, steep cut leaf or flower for five to ten minutes in boiling water.
- To make a decoction, boil cut root or bark for five to ten minutes on the stove.

Many people ask if the dosage of **dried herbs** should be different from **fresh herbs**. As the loss of chemicals in drying may balance the greater concentration due to loss of water, it is best to simply use the same amounts whether fresh or dry. Some herbs such as lemon balm, chamomile and basil taste better when fresh and are slightly more effective, but most herbs keep their medicinal qualities very well if dried carefully. Roots and barks often improve their taste with drying as they lose their acrid components and become sweeter.

Measurements
1ml = 1g
1 teaspoon = 5ml
1cup = 165ml
Tinctures are usually 1: 5, or 1 part herb to 5 parts
alcoholic liquid.

Doses for adults
Adults will usually require one to three cups a day of
herbal teas (whether infused or decocted), using one
teaspoon of herb per cup.

Adult doses of tincture vary according to the herbs used
in them. Usually half a teaspoon of single herb tinctures,
three times daily is required. With great care, you can get
80 drops onto a 5ml teaspoon, so you can work out your
dose that way too, and use the formula given above to
calculate a child's dose. The amount of alcohol is
negligible, but you can add the remedy to hot water and
allow some of the alcohol to evaporate if you wish.
Elderly people may require different doses, as body weight
falls, or if digestion isn't as good. Start with a lower dose
and work up if required.

Doses for children
Children require smaller doses. There are some formulae
which can be used, based on a child's age, for example:
divide the child's age by 20 to give the proportion of an
adult dose, i.e. 6 (years) divided by 20 = 3/10 adult dose.

You also have to take into account the child's body weight, giving less if a child is underweight for his/her age.

Common doses for teas are:

- a tablespoon of tea to a child under 5
- 1/2 cup for a child from 5 to 10 years
- a full cup from 11 years onwards.

Beatrice Potter seems to agree, as Peter Rabbit was given a large spoonful of chamomile tea after he had overeaten in Mr McGregor's garden!

Making your own formula

You can combine herbs in tincture or tea form to obtain a mixture of effects which will suit your individual needs. Start by choosing the actions that you want – for example relaxant, pain relieving, hormonal, and look for herbs which provide them. It is best to include no more than three or four herbs in one mixture, and with careful selection you can choose herbs with more than one action to match your requirements.

If you are using dried or fresh herbs to make teas, you should choose herbs which require the same sort of preparation (remember roots, barks and seeds need boiling, leaves and flowers need infusing). You will only need one teaspoon of your mix because herbs act synergistically as you have learnt already.

Tinctures

These have become very popular in Britain, both among herbalists and consumers. They are made by soaking finely chopped herbal material in an alcoholic liquid, about 70% proof. This could be brandy or vodka. Generally you use one part herb to five parts liquid, so 100g to 500ml. Chop the herbs as finely as possible and cover with the alcohol. Turn, shake or stir every day for ten days. This is to ensure that every particle of herb is in contact with alcohol, otherwise moulds may develop. After ten days, strain and squeeze out the remaining 'marc' through a clean piece of material. Keep the tincture you have made in a dry bottle with a tight stopper.

This can be used in place of herbal tea. Each teaspoon of tincture generally gives the effect of a small cup of tea. Sometimes herbal constituents are extracted better by alcohol, so it is a useful way of preserving herbs. In the past wines and vinegars were used. Their trace is found in the nursery rhyme Jack and Jill where 'Old Dame Dob did mend Jack's nob with vinegar and brown paper'.

It is obvious that these are much bigger doses than is often suggested on over-the-counter tincture bottles, where the manufacturer is more concerned with keeping the price and profit margin at an attractive level. Tinctures are more expensive than teas, and you should expect to pay between £3 and £5 for a week's supply.

Tincture of Lemon Balm

Ingredients
100g Lemon Balm
500ml vodka or brandy

Method
Chop herbs finely, cover with alcohol, shake or stir daily
for ten days, strain and bottle.

Herbal syrups

Herbs can be preserved in syrup but they are quite
difficult to make, as the proportion of sugar to herbal
material is crucial. They frequently go mouldy, however
carefully you measure. There are two methods, the first is
the simplest but only keeps for a few days.

Syrup recipe 1

Place chopped herb and sugar in 1cm layers in a clean,
dry jar, finishing with a sugar layer. Leave for one day –
you will find a syrup has formed. You can shake the jar
gently once a day until all the sugar has turned into syrup,
this may take three days but you can use the product
immediately.

Syrup recipe 2

Soak 4g of herb, finely chopped, in 56ml water for 12
hours. Strain and squeeze out the herbs. There should be
about 45ml liquid. Add 90g sugar, stir over heat until
dissolved, boil briefly, strain through a filter paper or
cloth. You should have about 100ml syrup. This must be

kept in a well stoppered bottle in a cool, dry, dark cupboard. The dose would usually be 1 teaspoon at a time for children, and a dessertspoon from 11 years onwards.

Pills

These come in two main varieties: pills and capsules. In both cases powdered herbs are used. Capsules are usually made of gelatine, although vegetarian ones can be obtained. Most are of a standard size, containing about 2g of herb. You can buy herbs ready powdered and fill your own capsules by hand. It's a very sneezy, time consuming business! Tablets are made by pressing powdered herbs into the required shape. You will need to add ingredients to make the dough stick together and the tablets hold their shape. Manufacturers usually use vegetable gums, but quite satisfactory tablets can be made at home using honey and arrowroot as binders. Pills can either be pinched off and rolled between the fingers or tablets cut by hand from dough rolled with a pin.

Buckwheat pills

Ingredients
2 tablespoons buckwheat flour
1 tablespoon arrowroot powder
4 teaspoons runny honey

Method
Knead all well together. Add more honey if required to achieve a malleable paste. Dust board with arrowroot, roll

out, cut to shape, dry on paper overnight.

Topical remedies

There are several forms in which herbs can be applied to the outside of your body. This is known as **topical application**. You need to remember a little bit about skin to understand how herbs reach their target when used in this way.

The Skin

Skin has several layers designed to keep water in (you suffer dehydration quickly if large areas of skin are broken) but allow moisture out when required to cool the body down by evaporation. It is covered with a cornified layer (dead cells) and wax. Blood vessels are very close to the surface, and they dilate when we are hot, to allow heat out by convection. They also dilate when we are emotionally stressed, so we flush with anger, embarassment, or affection. These blood vessels can constrict to conserve heat and sometimes, when we are very angry or upset, we become paler than our usual colour.

Fat underneath the skin keeps heat in by insulation and protects some areas from pressure (famously the bum!). Muscle is found underneath linings below the fatty layer. If you want to reach muscles, your topical applications must somehow get through the wax, cornified layer, fat and muscle linings first. Oily preparations do penetrate through these layers to some extent.

One way of increasing penetration is to soak the skin in water for a while. This can be done in the bath, in a steam room, or on small areas with a poultice or plaster. Belladonna plasters for back pain could still be bought in the chemist's until a few years ago. Most people have heard of anti-smoking and hormone patches. These use the same principle. Back to Old Dame Dob and her vinegar on brown paper!

Four ways of increasing absorption through the skin:

- bath
- steam
- poultice
- plaster.

Creams

Creams are more complicated to make. It would be easier to choose a favourite bland cream over the counter and add aromatic oils or tinctures as you wish. If you want to try a cream, try the following recipe:

Rosemary cream
Ingredients
8 parts oil
1 part beeswax
A few drops essential oil

Method
Gently heat oil and beeswax together in a bowl, set in a pan of water. When wax has melted, add essential oil. Pour into pots immediately.

Greasy ointments like this are generally not considered to be good for skin conditions such as eczema, where they inhibit healing and trap heat, but they are suitable for applying as muscle and joint rubs. Their advantage over liquid preparations is that they don't drip.

Massage oils

This option is useful if you want to use herbs from your garden. Simply pick a handful of fresh herbs, chop finely and cover loosely with any oil – almond, olive or even sunflower. Place the bowl of oil and herbs in a pan of water and put the lid on. Heat until simmering and leave on the lowest possible heat for 1-2 hours. A slow-pot can give ideal conditions for making infused oils as it maintains a constant, very low simmering temperature. Spices can also be used in infused oils.

There are many essential oils available now which save you the time involved in infusing plants in oil. The easiest way to apply these is in a carrier oil such as olive, almond or coconut. A few drops to a tablespoon will suffice.You can add a dash of chilli or ginger! Massaging increases blood flow to muscles and breaks down the tension in them. Rubbing creams and oils into small joints, such as fingers and toes, can give quite effective pain relief, and is particularly useful where the patient is unable to take any oral medication.

Baths

Essential oils can be added to the bath. Use a teaspoon of unscented bubble bath, or a tablespoon of milk to act as a dispersant. Relaxing bath salts are based on the same principle and available commercially, although they don't smell as nice as genuine essential oils. The pain relieving effect is limited, but a helpful contribution, especially at night before bed and there are no side-effects.

Plasters and poultices

These are used to apply steady heat or continued absorption of pain relieving or relaxing constituents to joints or muscles.

Plasters are made by melting one part of beeswax and two parts of vegetable oil, adding tincture or essential oil at the last minute. Soak a suitable sized cloth in the mix and spread out on a tray to cool and firm up. Apply to the body and cover in plastic or cling film (or paper!) and tie on with a bandage or some tight garment. The most common use is application to chest, back, abdomen and forehead. You could add a hot water bottle or hot towel wrap for extra comfort.

Poultices are similar to plasters, but consist of a 1cm thick layer of fresh or macerated herbs applied to the skin and covered with a piece of material. This was the earlier form of a plaster, but can still be immediate and effective.

Choosing, growing and storing herbs

Identifying herbs in the wild

It's important first of all to know that you have the right plant. Some botanical families include poisonous and edible plants which look very similar and can only be distinguished from each other by fine botanical detail. For example hemlock and valerian have subtle differences in stem and flower colouring. You could buy a field botany guide, as identification of plants is a great hobby, but it would be wiser not to select your remedies from the wild if you are a complete beginner.

Fortunately many of the most important medicinal herbs are garden favourites such as thyme, sage, rosemary, lemon balm and peppermint. Most people recognise them and they are pretty unmistakeable. Even where there are different varieties such as the Thymes and Mints, they have the same aroma and characteristics. It is better to choose the original sort for medicinal purposes rather than a variety, because it may be a more reliable source of the chemicals that you need for your remedy.

Choosing herbs

There is a system of naming plants which gives each one two Latin names – the family name comes first and has a capital letter, the individual name comes second written in lower case. The meaning is reversed in Latin, for example *Thymus vulgaris* means common thyme. This is the one you would use for cough medicine. Other types such as *Thymus aureus*, (golden thyme) or *Thymus serpillus* (creeping thyme) will do no harm, but they don't have as much aroma – in fact they put most of their energy into looking pretty! The same can be said for the many lovely varieties of achillea – a cottage garden flower related to yarrow (*Achillea officinalis*). The word *officinalis* in a plant's name means it was known to be used medicinally in the seventeenth century or before. You will need to specify both names when you are buying seeds or plants from nurseries. Addresses of reliable firms are given on page 138.

Growing herbs

Many of the herbs mentioned in this book can be grown in British gardens, some can be grown in pots or window ledges. Growing herbs is a very relaxing and rewarding hobby. Although most aromatic herbs originate in the warm Mediterranean countries, they will do fine in a sunny spot in any garden soil, even on London clay. They do prefer well drained (slightly dry) soil, so adding grit and compost will help them along.

If you are growing from seed you will need to start them off in pots first on a window ledge or in a greenhouse. To sow seeds really successfully, you should buy John Innes compost number one. This contains lots of sand and fine grit, so that water runs through quickly and the seed doesn't sit in its own tiny puddle of water, which causes a fungal growth gardeners call damping off.

When you have a small stem with two leaves, pull it up gently and plant in a pot with John Innes number two compost. This has more soil, so that fine roots can spread and take in water – it also contains a little more nutrient to feed the growing plant. When your plant is about 10 cm tall or has a few branches, it's time to plant it in a sunny spot or container, using John Innes number three. 'John Innes' is a type of compost, not a brand name, so you can ask for it at any garden nursery.

Planting out

Locate your herbs in the south west corner of your garden if possible. Herbs don't need feeding or watering once they have extended their roots into the garden soil (after about a week), but containers will need to be watered as they dry out continually. You can even grow herbs in hanging baskets. You can use multi-purpose compost, but you run a much greater risk of damping-off and losing seed before they even grow, which can mean a whole growing year lost. If your plants don't succeed in one spot in your garden, move them! Just dig up enough soil around the plant to ensure minimum root disturbance and put them in somewhere else. Experiment to see what works. There are plenty of herbs to choose from, so find one that suits your garden or space.

- Choose a sunny spot.
- Add grit to improve drainage.
- Start tender plants under glass.
- Water pots and baskets daily.
- Move plants if they aren't happy.

Choosing the right part of the plant

It's important to know which part of the plant you need if you are going to make your own herbal remedies. Flowers, leaves, roots, bark and berries are commonly used but sometimes one part of a plant is edible whereas another part is poisonous. We eat the tuberous root of the potato but avoid the berries and we eat rhubarb stems but not the leaves. Comfrey root stores too many alkaloids, which can damage the liver, whereas they are barely present in the leaf. It is common to find stems in with leaves in herbs sold over the counter, as it is difficult to separate them when preparing herbs on a large scale. If you are preparing your own, you should take the trouble to rub the leaves off the stems as your remedy will be stronger without this inert woody matter.

Harvesting herbs

Choosing the right time to harvest is also important. It helps you to get the best quality of herbs in terms of the chemical constituents.

- Leaves are picked just before flowers develop.
- Flowers are picked as they come out.
- Berries as they become fully ripe, while they are still smooth and shiny.
- Bark and stem is stripped in the late spring from new branches.
- Roots are dug up in early autumn before the first frosts. Pick on a dry day, and scrub roots immediately after digging.

Storing herbs

Most plants can be used fresh, but it is more convenient to dry them for use all the year round.

Drying herbs

The rules for drying herbs are: as cool, fast, dark and dry as possible, with as much air circulating around the individual herbs as can be allowed. The best way for home preservation is to hang up small bunches of herbs, loosely tied, in a dark room or shed. A washing-line strung across the attic is ideal, hanging up in the kitchen will cause most of the colour and aroma to be lost before they dry.

Large roots should be chopped before drying, as they will prove too tough for the knife otherwise. They can be spread out in a single layer on newspapers. The newspapers should be changed when they feel very damp.

Herbal material is ready to store when it is cracking dry. This is a matter of experience, usually leaves will simply not leave their stems until they are thoroughly dry. Roots should snap briskly or fail to bend under pressure. Berries usually give a little under thumb pressure, they are slow to dry – moulds develop if there is too much moisture so gentle heat (airing cupboard level) is helpful. When thoroughly dry herbs should be stored in cool, dark, dry, airless conditions because sunlight destroys colour, air removes flavour and water causes moulds. Tin boxes are ideal, however plastic tubs and glass jars are OK provided they are kept in a cupboard.

- Hang leaves on branches upside down.
- Spread roots out in a single layer.
- Dry as fast as possible in a cool, dark, airy place.
- Ready when cracking dry.
- Keep in cool, dark, dry, airless conditions.

~ 6 ~

Using nutrition for bone, joint and muscle health

Achieving a balanced diet

Nearly everyone agrees that what we eat affects our health. Most complementary health practitioners believe that our diet affects the way we experience diseases as well. In Britain research into food was started during World War II and was continued by the Ministry of Agriculture and Fisheries with help from the Medical Research Council. They produced guidelines on what people need to eat to make them healthy. These are called the **minimum daily requirements** and they cover the main nutrients needed by the human body. In America the USDA (United States Department of Agriculture) funds a similar programme, and their books are widely used in Britain.

It is a mistake to look at single nutrients as being a cure for specific conditions, as almost all body processes require a broad range of nutrients to keep them running smoothly. It is true that bones require calcium for strength but they also need protein, phosphates and some magnesium, as well as a good blood supply and nerve transmission, which in their turn have special nutrient needs.

All human cells need sugar as a fuel to perform their vital functions, osteoblasts and osteoclasts (bone makers and breakers) are no exception. Muscle uses sugar for fuel as well as calcium and potassium to contract and relax. Salt (sodium) plays an essential role in getting calcium into muscle fibre cells and potassium is vital to maintain the correct amount of salt in the body. All these processes are dependent on each other and on a balanced state of nutrients in the body. This is the state of health which the herbalist tries to restore with herbal medicines and wholistic dietary advice. It is usual to divide food up into seven different categories and we should aim to eat something in each category every day.

You could use these categories to design a food diary or plan your eating for a week.

- **Protein** – cheese, meat, beans, nuts, fish
- **Starch** – bread, potatoes, pasta, roots, rice, grains
- **Vitamin A** – green, orange and yellow vegetables
- **Vitamin B** – meat, wholegrains
- **Vitamin C** – fresh fruit and green vegetables
- **Vitamin D** – fish oil and sunlight
- **Vitamin E** – wholegrains and seeds
- **Vitamin P** – also known as bioflavonoids (fresh fruit and vegetables)
- **Minerals** – calcium, potassium, sodium, magnesium, zinc, phosphorus, found in vegetable and animal foods
- **Trace elements** – cobalt, copper etc , found in vegetable and animal foods

- **Fibre** (indigestible parts of vegetables and grains)
- **Fat** (butter, cooking oil, margarine).

Daily requirements for nutrients

These vary according to age and occupation (whether you have an active or sedentary job). Here, we have taken the figures for sedentary workers. You can use these tables to understand information given on labelling of supplements

- 1mg = one thousandth of 1g , 1μg = 1 millionth of 1g

	Men 35-64	Women 18-54
kcals	2,400	2,150
protein	60g	54g
calcium	500mg	500mg
iron	10mg	12mg
vitamin A	750μg	750μg
thiamin (vitamin B$_1$)	1mg	.8mg
riboflavin (vitamin B$_2$)	1.6mg	1.3mg
niacin (vitamin B)	18mg	15mg
vitamin C	30mg	30mg
vitamin D	10μg if no sunlight available	10μg if no sunlight available

Women's needs vary to a greater extent than men's because of changes taking place during pregnancy, breastfeeding, the monthly menstrual cycle and menopause. British guidelines suggest that women over 55 take fewer calories (1,900kcals) and less iron (10mg) daily. The lower iron intake is suggested because there will be no monthly losses due to menstruation and the smaller calorie intake reflects metabolic changes after the menopause.

American researchers give us figures for some of the other vital nutrients which apply to both men and women.

vitamin K	70-140µg
biotin (vitamin B)	100-200µg
pantothenin (vitamin B)	4-7mg
potassium	1,875-562 mg
phosphorus	700-800mg
sodium	1,100-3,300
chloride	1,700-5,100

Canadian guidelines complete the picture, with daily requirements for men and women between 25 and 49 and recommendations for the over 50s (blank means no change).

	Men	(over 50)	Women	(over 50)
vitamin E	9mg	7mg	6mg	
folacin (vitamin B)	220µg		175µg	190µg
pyridoxine (vitamin B_{12})	2µg		2µg	
magnesium	250mg		200mg	210mg
calcium	800mg		700mg	800mg
iodine	160µg		160µg	
zinc	9mg		8mg	

It's interesting to note that Canadian researchers think we need a lot more daily calcium than their British counterparts. This is because they recommend a much higher protein intake which causes greater loss of calcium from the body. You may need to take this into account when you are looking at labels on vitamin and minerals supplements.

Other minerals considered essential for daily nutrition are chromium, selenium, molybdenum, copper, manganese and fluoride. The intakes for these are generally very small figures from .2 to .5μg. These are called trace elements.

The guidelines presented above are based on the amounts needed to stop you developing a deficiency condition, such as scurvy (which develops when you don't get enough vitamin C). Some nutritionists think you need more than these if you have certain diseases, but this is a very undefined area, with lots of claims motivated by the desire to sell products. Although, as stated before, general health is achieved by eating a balance of all necessary nutrients, some are more clearly associated with bone health than others. We will explore the role of these nutrients in maintaining healthy muscles, joints and bones below.

Protein (daily requirement – 60g)

Essential for muscle and bone strength.

You will find 60g of protein in	Normal portion	Gives approx. % daily need
200g cheddar cheese	50g	25%
300g white meat (350g red meat)	75g	33%
400g fish	100g	25%
400g peanuts	50g	12.5%
500g kidney beans	50g	10%
720g tofu	75g	9.5%
2 litres of milk	150ml	7.5%
10 eggs	1 egg	10%
900g barley	50g	5%
1,000g bread	100g (2 medium slices)	10%

It's important to 'read between the lines' when looking at figures like these. You could have larger portions of beans, or (like ancient Britons) eat barley instead of rice. This would give you bigger portions and much higher values for your daily intake. If you rely on cheese for your protein, you have to be aware that it contains as much fat per 10g as it does protein. Bread has a lot of starch as well as protein, and you may be surprised to know that brown bread has no more protein than white. Fish has a lot of water in it, which is why we take a bigger portion by weight. Peanuts appear to be as good as fish, weight for weight, but they contain a lot of fat.

You also need to know that protein is made up of 22 amino acids. Some foods have these in equal quantities, like eggs, cheese, fish and meat, whereas other foods (such as beans and grains) don't. This can be offset by combining certain foods to provide a balance. Beans on toast is a famous example, rice and peas is another. The bean family does have the benefit of giving us fibre and minerals, which are low in animal foods, as well as being much cheaper to produce and buy.

Ways of adding protein to your daily diet

The percentage increase is based on the normal portions given in the table above.

Food	Percentage of daily requirement
egg or baked beans for breakfast	10%
egg in bread (brioche, delicious!)	6%
ground almond thickening	6%
peanut butter as sauce (Thai style)	6%
pearl barley instead of rice	6%
sweet bean sauce (chinese style)	10%
ground nuts in pastry	6%
grated cheese as dressing	12.5%
egg in puddings	10%
milk in puddings	7.5%
beans in soup	10%
grilled bacon or sausage for breakfast	16.5%
extra protein in sandwich	up to 16.5%
egg noodles	6%

Minerals

Calcium

Daily requirement 500g. Used to give rigidity to bone.

You will find 500mg calcium in	Normal portion	Gives approx. % daily need
50g dried milk	10g	20%
70g cheddar cheese	50g	66%
100g tinned sardines	50g	50%
200g watercress	25g	12.5%
200g figs	25g	12.5%
250g almonds	50g	25%
500ml milk	150ml	32%
500g white bread (1,000g wholemeal)	100g	25%
600g spinach	50g	8%
600g kidney beans	50g	8%

It may surprise you to find that meat, eggs and fish contain almost no calcium (it's the bones in tinned sardines which provide your calcium!). White bread only has calcium because it is added by law in Britain to white flour but not to wholemeal.

All dark green leaf vegetables contain significant amounts of calcium. Parsley is similar to watercress, kale and broccoli are similar to spinach. Most nuts contain the same amount of calcium as almonds.

You will have no problem easily reaching your calcium

requirements if you take milk and cheese in your diet. If you are unable or unwilling to take milk products, you will have to work a lot harder at balancing your diet for calcium.

Ways of adding calcium to your diet

The percentage increase is based on normal portions given in the table above.

Food	Percentage of daily requirement
white bread sandwiches	25%
cheese sauce	53%
grated cheese dressing	33%
beans on white toast	33%
ground almond thickening (Indian style)	20%
parsley sauce (milk)	32.5%
white cheese in curry (last minute, Indian style)	33%
cheese cubes in salad	33%
extra milk powder in milk dishes	20%
calcium fortified soya milk	10%

Some factors influence the amount of calcium our body can absorb, increasing or decreasing the amount we take in.

Increase calcium absorption	Reduced calcium absorption
acids (citrus drinks, tomato sauce)	tannins (tea)
phosporus (cheese, sardines, quality milk chocolate!)	fibre (bran, beans)
vitamin D	phytic acids (bran, non-yeast bread)
digestive herbs	high protein diets

Yeast fermentation uses up most of the phytic acid in bread, so helps to maximise absorption of calcium. Unfortunately, modern factory breadmaking methods replace yeast with carbon dioxide. You may wish to make your own or find a local baker who still uses yeast in his bread. All these factors only exert their effects at or near to mealtimes, so you should drink your juice with a meal and you can still have your cup of tea, but not straight after a meal!

Potassium

Daily requirement 1,875mg. Used to relax and contract muscles, exchanges with sodium.

You will find 1,875mg potassium in	Normal portion	Gives approx. % daily need
165g haricot beans	50g	10%
170g dried peaches	25g	16%
175g parsley	10g	6%
200g almonds	50g	25%
275g peanuts	50g	20%

275g potato	100g	40%
600g dark chocolate	50g	8%
850g bananas	100g	12.5%

You can see that dried fruit and beans are a very good source of potassium. You could substitute others with the same value, such as kidney beans or pears. It is really important to retain the water you soaked the dried beans in, as two thirds of the potassium is absorbed into it, so rinse them first and use the soaking water for cooking. Meat, fish and cheese have very small amounts of potassium, so aren't listed here. Mashed potato has one third the amount of potassium as baked (due to losses in cooking water) and bananas contain a lot of starch along with the potassium.

Ways of adding potassium to your daily diet

Based on normal portions given above.

- Dried fruit and nuts instead of biscuits
- Rich fruit cake instead of doughnuts
- Beans in stew or meat dishes
- Beans in soup
- Parsley dressings and sauces
- Thicken sauces with ground almonds
- Marzipan instead of sweets.

Phosphorus

Daily requirement 700mg. Part of the bonding structures which give bone rigidity and strength.

You will find 700mg phosphorus in	Normal portion	Gives approx. % daily need
600g pumpkin seed	25g	45%
90g sesame seed	20g	18%
150g cheddar cheese	50g	33%
150g sardines	50g	33%
150g kidney beans	50g	33%
150g cocoa	10g	6%
250g haricot beans	50g	20%
350g white meat (500g red meat)	75g	25%
400g mushrooms	50g	12.5%
500g plain chocolate	50g	10%

Phosphorus is found in largest amounts in seeds and nuts but is also found in animal protein.If you cook beans carefully, retaining all water, they can provide satisfactory daily amounts. Nuts have high amounts of fat, so you will need to cut fat elsewhere if you rely on these for nutrients.

Ways of adding phosphorus to your daily diet

Based on normal portions given above.

- Seeds in bread mix
- Seeds on bread rolls

- Tahini (sesame butter) in spreads
- Peanut butter on toast
- Bean soup for lunch
- Real cocoa for drinks and cakes.

Magnesium

Daily requirement 250mg. Enables muscles to relax, essential for energy use in muscles.

You will find 250mg magnesium in	Normal portion	Gives approx. % daily need
70g sunflower seed	25g	40%
75g sesame seed	25g	33%
75g almonds	50g	66%
100g brazil nuts	50g	50%
100g cashews (roasted)	25g	25%
140g peanuts	50g	35%
200g haricot beans	50g	25%
240g tofu	50g	18%

Nuts and seeds are the best sources of magnesium, followed by the bean family whose members all provide important amounts of this mineral. You can substitute others for the ones listed here. You will need to be careful with other fats in your diet if you eat a lot of nuts. They provide us with mainly monosaturated fats, which aren't quite as 'good' as unsaturated fats. Magnesium is also found in smaller amounts in green vegetables, so including more than one helping per day in your diet will contribute a little to your magnesium intake.

Ways of adding magnesium to your daily diet

Based on normal portions given above.

- Nut mix instead of biscuits
- Nut loaf instead of meat
- Seeds in bread mix
- Tofu in stir fry or curry
- Ground nuts in pastry
- Bean soup for lunch (again!)
- Nuts in cakes.

Vitamins

Vitamin D

Daily requirement 10µg.

You will find 10µg Vitamin D in	Normal portion	Gives approx. % daily need
4g cod liver oil	4ml	100%
50g oily fish	100g	200%
75g tinned salmon	50g	66%
125g tinned sardines	50g	40%
150g margarine (made with fish oil)	10g (in baking)	6%
200ml evaporated milk	75ml	38%

Vitamin D[1] is found naturally only in animal foods.

Vitamin D^2 , which works almost as well as D^1, can be manufactured from small amounts (.03-.06 per 100g) in legumes such as mung beans, lentils and chickpeas. These are not useful amounts for the human body to use but provide a vegetarian source for commercial supplements.

Humans normally obtain vitamin D from sunlight's action on their skin. Pale-skinned people need one hour's exposure of their face to midday, cloudless sun for their daily requirement. Dark-skinned people need three hours in the same conditions. Not so easy in a cloudy northern climate! Worries about ozone holes and skin cancers have complicated things and doctors are busy arguing about how long you can stay in the sun. It seems that half-an-hour, face, arms and legs will do the trick, so it might be important for people who are shy about uncovering their body to have somewhere private to do this.

It is also really important to know that you can overdose on vitamin D if you take too much fish oil. Halibut oil is many times more concentrated than cod liver oil, so you must never confuse the two.

Increasing daily intake of vitamin D

- Walk or cycle to work
- Eat lunch outside
- Sit in the garden after work
- Buy vegetarian, vitamin D enriched margarine
- More legumes!

- Oily fish (sprats, mackerel, salmon, sardines)
- Hard margarine in baking
- Short spells of sunbathing in shorts or shift!

Vitamin E

Vitamin E is found in vegetable oil and wholegrains. It prevents the oxidation (destruction) of essential fatty acids, so may help to protect secretory membranes such as synovial and mucus membranes. Research has shown that Vitamin E supplements alleviate some leg cramps (at night-time and on walking) although the method of action isn't clear. Heat destroys it, but it is stored in the body for a long time, so you could build up a supply in the summer salad months.

Remember!

Minerals are stored in the bones and vitamin D is stored in the body so you won't go short if you miss your target once a week, as long as you make it up over the next week. Excesses aren't good for you, and over-emphasis on one mineral or vitamin can cause imbalances in others, resulting in muscle cramps, twitching, or weakness.

Fats

As we find out more about fats, we discover that essential fatty acids (those we cannot make for ourselves) are needed in all sorts of body processes. They are found in polyunsaturated fats and there are three of them, called linoleic, linolenic and arachidonic acid. They may be used up in inflammatory diseases as they are the building blocks for immune system messengers. They are also a vital part of secretory cell walls. These produce important linings such as the synovial membrane, which lubricates joints. It is possible that extra plant oils may protect joints from deterioration. You should increase these oils in your diet, at the expense of animal fats which can't be used for anything but insulation and energy. Liquid oils contain the most polyunsaturated fats, they are all found only in plants. There aren't yet any recommended daily requirements for essential fats.

Plants which give us poly-unsaturated fats

- Evening Primrose
- grapeseed
- hemp
- maize (corn)
- nuts
- olive
- rape seed
- sesame
- soya
- Starflower (borage)
- sunflower

You could aim at 10ml daily of any of these oils, varying them to include as many as you can in your diet, as each contains different proportions of essential fatty acids.

Ways of adding essential fatty acids to your daily diet

- Add a teaspoon of oil to your meal at the end of cooking
- Take a little French dressing or mayonnaise
- Use vegetable oil spread instead of butter
- Make cakes with plant oil (carrot cake, chocolate cake are particularly good.

Other useful nutrients

Vitamin A

Vitamin A is found in dark green leaf, orange and yellow vegetables. It is vital for the growth of bone, so essential for children. It is stored in the liver for up to a year, excess causes damage, which is why it is better to rely on salad, rather than juices.

Zinc

Zinc is required to release vitamin A from storage and to process essential fatty acids in the body. It is mainly found in meat, shellfish, eggs and wholegrains. Cow's milk protein reduces its absorption, wine increases it.

Making room for change

If you want to make room for these extra nutrients you may need to look carefully at the day's eating, to see if there is too much carbohydrate (potatoes, flour, sugar, sweet roots – eg yam and casava) or fat. These fill you up, but don't provide the essential nutrients in sufficient quantities. It's no good having all the right foods in the house if you've filled up on starch and don't feel like eating them. Try to avoid snacks between meals and get the 'essentials' on the plate first.

One way of changing your eating habits is to make a food diary, like the one shown on page 128. It can be interesting and very revealing! Use the nutrition tables above to assign your eating to the right rows.This model is not meant to give you detailed information on meeting daily requirements, but to give you an idea of balance. Many herbalists use detailed dietary analysis in their consultations. The first column is filled in to show you how it can be used. If you assume that each entry is a normal portion, you will be able to see roughly how near you get to your daily requirement of each item.

The example given is a very typical diet and is very high in fat and starch, with no fibre, as the bread and pasta used is white. Note that the main ingredient in most soft drinks is sugar, so this has been entered in the starch column. Labels on packaged food tell you which is the greatest ingredient, so you can tell where to assign it.

	Monday	Tuesday	Wednesday	Thursday	Friday	Saturday	Sunday
Protein	Tuna Cheese						
Fat	Butter Cheese Cake						
Starch	Bread Pasta Crisps Cake Cordial						
Vitamins	Orange Juice Tomatoes						
Minerals	Cheese						
Trace Elements	Tea						
Fibre							

A food diary

❧ 7 ❧

Case histories

The remedies given to these patients were in tincture form, usually 5ml, 3 times daily, the herbs were prescribed in equal parts(about 20ml of each in a weekly amount of 100ml). To make a tea mix you would take equal parts and pre-mix, then use a heaped teaspoon (5ml) of your mix, 3 times daily.

Case 1 Arthritis and anxiety

Miss H, a 29 year old office worker, noticed pain in her legs and arms, wrists and ankles when sitting for any length of time at work. It was worse in the evening and especially bad ten days or more before a period. It began soon after she had stopped taking the contraceptive pill. The stiffness in her joints was increasing and she noticed puffiness under the eyes as well as back pain. She was also suffering panic attacks which caused difficulty in breathing together with sharp chest pains. Her doctor had arranged a heart check-up and this proved normal. Miss H had recently taken on a new job which involved supervising staff and longer hours.

On examination her joints were not swollen, but tender to finger pressure. her joints were a little stiff but she could move them all freely. During her first consultation we discussed her priorities for treatment, and she decided that pain relief and relaxation were most important, as this would enable her to 'get on top of her job'. Water retention appeared to be a feature of her hormone cycle which made matters worse, so we chose herbs with secondary diuretic properties where possible.

Her remedy was fairly simple and worked well, relieving anxiety and arthritic symptoms.:

- Celery seed – anti-inflammatory, diuretic, mild relaxant
- Burdock – cleansing, diuretic
- Willowbark – anti-inflammatoy, pain reliever, mild oestrogenic
- Valerian – major relaxant.

Miss H took this treatment for several months, until she felt confident and less 'stretched' at work. Then she moved onto a routine of taking diuretic herb teas in the second half of her cycle, which prevented pain from re-occurring.

Case 2 Severe rheumatoid arthritis and immobility

Mrs B, a retired cashier of 60 who had suffered rheumatoid arthritis for years, had a sudden attack of severe pain and swelling in all joints shortly after her husband died of a heart attack at 63. She had become completely immobile, being unable to get out of bed without help. She hadn't left the house in two years relying on daily nursing care for washing and brought-in meals. She took a number of other medications and had noticed a rash appearing when she took aspirin. She also suffered from constipation, partly because of immobility and partly due to her pain-relieving medication.

Mrs B's priority was to improve mobility and relieve her constipation. Her joints were cold and very swollen, with considerable distortion in all her fingers, she was unable even to turn her head. Her diet diary revealed that she ate white bread and her meals contained little vegetable content. We chose non-salicylate pain relievers (to avoid exacerbating her aspirin based rash) and cleansing herbs with laxative qualities as well as muscle relaxants to help mobility of digestive and body muscles.
Her remedy consisted of:

- Guaiac – cleansing, anti-inflammatory
- Celery seed – diuretic, anti-inflammatory
- Devil's claw – non salicylate, anti-inflammatory pain-reliever
- Wild Yam – muscle relaxant.

Wintergreen oil was used to rub into the wrists and fingers, which provided extra pain relief without systemic absorption of salicylates.

One month later there was a small improvement in mobility of hands, neck and knees, noticed by the patient and the physiotherapist. Although the progress was slow, by the end of six months Mrs B was able to say that she was far more comfortable when taking herbal medicine than before, and was able to take fewer pain relievers, which resulted in better digestion (she also changed over to wholemeal bread). She would have benefited from an extended stay in a continental-style hydro, where mineral baths and dietary changes could have made a big contribution to improvement in mobility.

Case 3 Arthritis, stomach ulcer and heart problems

Mr G, a 58-year-old ex-builder, had recently suffered a heart attack, was very overweight, with a stomach ulcer caused by aspirin use for arthritis in hips, feet, hands and knees. The joints in his feet and hands were a little enlarged but not hot. His life was very stressful and he was currently unable to work. He took beta-blockers and antacids.

Mr G had suffered a major shock in discovering how unhealthy he was. He was trying hard to change his diet, but found it difficult. He agreed that stress and anxiety were contributing to his heart problems and continued indigestion. His priorities were relief from pain and joint-swelling, heart health, digestive improvement and relaxation.

His remedy was:

- Celery seed – diuretic, anti-inflammatory
- Hawthorn – heart tonic

- Dandelion root – digestive tonic, cleanser
- Dandelion leaf – potassium-rich diuretic cleanser
- Passionflower – relaxant, relieves high blood pressure
- Slippery elm tablets were prescribed for instant relief from heartburn and longer-term healing for the stomach.

This brought relief to pain in knees, hands and feet after two weeks. Mr. C said he felt much more able to deal with the many problems besetting him. His blood pressure came down a little, and he continued to have his heart monitored at regular hospital visits. We discussed Weight Watchers, and he was assured that it wasn't only for women!

Case 4 Arthritis, elderly health care and angina

Mrs D, an 80-year-old housewife, suffered from pain in knees and shoulders, the left knee being swollen. She noticed a tight feeling in her calves when walking, her shoulder pain was worse at night and she had angina, for which she occasionally took medication. She also took tablets for her high blood pressure. Her husband was frail and ill, needing lots of hospital visits. Mrs D was worried about the consequences for him if she were to become ill or immobile. Her priorities were mobility and heart health. We chose herbs which nourished heart muscle, kept blood vessels relaxed and reduced painful swelling in joints. Digestive tonics were used to improve overall health and energy.

Her remedy consisted of:

- Willowbark – anti-inflammatory pain reliever
- Celery seed – anti-inflammatory, diuretic
- Dandelion root – diuretic, digestive tonic
- Dandelion leaf – potassium-rich diuretic
- Cramp Bark – muscle relaxant, relieves high blood pressure and anginal cramps.

Mrs D called this her life-saver!

Case 5 Arthritis and indigestion

Mr F, a 54 -year-old electrician, had pain in all his joints, especially shoulders. He frequently suffered from wind and colic.

This remedy brought complete relief from shoulder pain by the next visit:

- Dandelion root – liver tonic
- Celery seed – anti-inflammatory and diuretic cleansing herb
- Willowbark – anti-inflammatory and pain reliever
- Prickly Ash – circulatory tonic
- Chilli (a few drops) – circulatory tonic
- Cramp Bark – muscle relaxant
- Lemon Balm tea – mental relaxant and general digestive tonic.

Case 6 Rheumatism in teenagers

Miss O, a 15-year-old schoolgirl, had experienced pains in her legs since she was 13. She started having light-sensitive headaches two months before and was having very heavy periods. She was taking antibiotics for acne. Her priorities were to replace the antibiotics, improve skin and relieve muscular pain and headaches. Iron tonics were included to offset blood loss from heavy periods.
Her remedy consisted of:

- Feverfew – to relieve blood vessel spasm and migraine, anti-inflammatory
- Oregon grape – cleansing, liver tonic to clear skin
- Cramp Bark – muscle relaxant for period and leg pains
- Nettles – iron tonic, anti-inflammatory
- Ginger (a few drops) – circulatory tonic.

Miss O's symptoms gradually disappeared over two months.

Case 7 Rheumatism and nervous tension

This has been included to show how one can underestimate the power of nervous tension!

Mr M, a 35-year-old pavier, had painful muscular tension in neck and shoulders, heartburn and wind. His contracting work and mortgage caused him great worry. We decided that his work was causing muscular and digestive problems (lifting , bending and kneeling all day). His first remedy was:

- Cramp Bark –muscle relaxant ·
- Hops – digestive relaxant
- Meadowsweet – antacid, anti-spasmodic, anti-inflammatory.

This resulted in much better digestion but no relief from pain in shoulders. His remedy was changed to:

- Damiana (an anti-depressant male tonic)
- Hops – digestive tonic
- Skullcap – nervine relaxant.

This worked a treat! Obviously the mainly peripheral relaxants of the first remedy hadn't addressed the root of the problem.

Sources and resources

Nutrition – further reading

MAFF Manual of Nutrition (HMSO). A brief guide to the contents of major foods and dietary guidelines with daily requirements. This book was used by every home economics student and teacher from the 1950s until the 1980s when cookery and nutrition became design and labelling!

Identifying herbs – further reading

The Concise British Flora Publisher, W. Keble-Martin (Ebury Press). The author was a vicar who spent all his spare time painting wild flowers. This is a remarkable book which captures the essence of each flower and plant. Better than photos for identifying difficult to recognise subjects. Not easy to use, as the plants are arranged in families, but worth persevering.

Exercise

The British Wheel of Yoga, 25 Jermyn St, Sleaford, Lincolnshire NG34 7RU. Tel: (01529) 303233. The main association for yoga teachers and those interested in yoga. Hatha yoga is the type which has most general application – it is yoga for health. This is mainly what you will find being taught in evening classes and lunchtime sessions. It consists of a series of tone and stretch exercises which have been developed over thousands of years in India. Most teachers include some exercises from other strands of yoga as these are more directly designed to relax the mind and are associated with meditation. Some people with strong religious faiths are afraid that yoga involves taking up a mystic religion. This isn't true – the meditations are designed to make you aware of your mind and enable you to empty it. They can be performed by members of any religious group.

Seeds

King's Seeds, Monk's Farm, Coggeshall Road, Kelvedon, Essex CO5 9PG. Tel: (01376) 572456. Previously Suffolk herbs, this is the only company in Britain selling a wide variety of wild flower and herb seeds.

Samuel Dobie and Son, Long Rd, Paignton, Devon TQ4 7SX. Tel: (01803) 696444. Dobie's Seeds sell a wide range of flower and vegetable seeds, with a good selection of culinary herbs.

Seeing herbs

The Chelsea Physic Garden, Royal Hospital Walk (entrance in Cheyne Walk), London. (Sloane Square tube). Probably the best collection in Britain, begun in the seventeenth century, brilliant teas and cakes, exquisite pleasure to walk round. Open Sundays from 2pm and some weekdays. Run by volunteers (who make the cakes!). Tel: (0207) 352 5646.

Buying dried herbs and preparations

Alban Mills Herbs, 38, Sandridge Rd, St Albans AL1 4AS.
Tel: (01727) 858243. *www.lsgmills@care4free.net*
A very large range of medicinal and culinary herbs and
spices, creams, oils, syrups, tablets, toiletries and essential
oils. Small amounts no problem.

Gardening

The Henry Doubleday Research Association has its own
seed catalogue, run by Chase Organics, and a magazine
for subscribers which gives advice on organic gardening
and news of organic projects in Britain and abroad. E-
mail: *membership@hdra.org.uk* Tel: (024) 76 303517.

Gardener's Question Time, 2pm Sunday Radio 4, repeated
in the day-time during the week, has been offering
gardening advice from a panel of experts to live audiences
for generations. *Gardener's World*, 8.30 BBC2, still offers a
designer-free zone of real gardening.

Consulting herbalists

The National Institute of Medical Herbalists (NIMH), 56
Longbrook St, Exeter, Devon EX46AH. Tel: (01392)
426022. *www.btinternet.com/~nimh/*. The National Institute
of Medical Herbalists was established in 1864 to promote
training and standards in herbal medicine. It is the oldest
body of professional herbalists in the world. Members
train for four years to a Bsc in Herbal Medicine, which

involves herbal pharmacology, medical sciences and pharmacognosy (the science of recognising herbal compounds and materials).

Representatives of the NIMH sit on government committees and are involved in decisions on the safety of herbal medicines in Britain and Europe.

Counselling and talking therapies

Self-help books are abundant. You will need to read more than one to get an idea of the different sorts of talking therapies. Contact How To Books for a catalogue.

Patient support groups

These are extremely useful for sharing problems and solutions. Ask in your local library for the *Directory of Associations* which contains all national associations and is updated annually. The current secretarial address for the Arthritis Association is listed there.

List of herbs within their applications

Anti-inflammatories

Black cohosh
Celery seed
Devil's claw
Feverfew
Ginger
Guaiac
Liquorice
Meadowsweet
Poplar
Willowbark

Cleansing herbs

Burdock
Celery
Dandelion
Kelp
Nettles
Sarsaparilla
Yellow dock

Pain relievers

Passionflower
Poppy
Silver birch
St John's wort
Wild lettuce
Wintergreen

Relaxants

Black cohosh
Chamomile
Cowslips
Cramp bark
Kava- kava
Lemon balm
Limeflowers
Passionflower
Skullcap
St John's wort
Valerian
Vervein
Wild yam

Circulatory tonics

Chilli
Garlic
Ginger
Horseradish
Mustard
Prickly ash

Rubefacient oils

Cedarwood
Juniper
Lavender
Pine
Rosemary
Thyme
Wintergreen

Digestive tonics

Chilli
Galangal
Ginger
Horseradish
Lemon balm
Rosemary
Sage
Thyme

Healing herbs

Comfrey

General Index